# THE Nursing Mother's Companion

# THE *Nursing Mother's Companion*

REVISED EDITION

## *Kathleen Huggins*

Foreword by Ruth A. Lawrence
Photographs by Harriette Hartigan

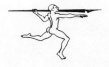

THE HARVARD COMMON PRESS
Harvard and Boston, Massachusetts

The Harvard Common Press
535 Albany Street
Boston, Massachusetts 02118

Printed in the United States of America

**Library of Congress Cataloging-in-Publication Data**
Huggins, Kathleen.
    The nursing mother's companion / Kathleen
Huggins ; foreword by Ruth A. Lawrence. — Rev. ed.
        p.    cm.
    ISBN 1-55832-025-3 : $16.95. — ISBN
1-55832-026-1 : $9.95
    1. Breast feeding.  I. Title.
RJ216.H845  1990
649'.33—dc20                                    90-38863

Drawings by Susan Aldridge
Cover design by Jackie Schuman
Text design by Linda Ziedrich

10  9  8  7  6  5

*To the nursing mothers of San Luis Obispo,
who have been my teachers*

# Contents

# Foreword

Centuries ago few women faced decisions about how to feed their babies: the newborn's only means of survival was mother's milk. Today, however, there are safe alternatives to nursing, and so a woman needs to think about how she wishes to feed her baby and what method is really best for them both. If she decides to nurse her baby as her ancestors did theirs, she must make an effort to learn how. Breastfeeding is the physiologic continuation of the normal reproductive cycle, and babies are born knowing how to find the nipple and to suck; their mothers, however, do not instinctively know how to nurse. Many women today have never seen a baby breastfed and have little access to experienced nursing mothers. Today's mothers have to learn what to do.

An expectant mother must first learn about alternative feeding methods so she can make an informed choice. With this book Kathleen Huggins helps the mother through the decision-making process by providing sound information about the practical advantages of breastfeeding, its importance to a baby's health, and the very special emotional rewards it offers both mother and baby.

As a woman progresses through her pregnancy and makes preparations for her baby, she may wonder how she should also prepare for breastfeeding. Inexperienced though well-meaning friends may offer abundant but conflicting advice. This book, on the contrary, provides sensible guidelines for preparing to breastfeed, as well as an explanation of the process by which nature prepares the breast for nursing. Understanding how the breast functions prepares a woman for the physiologic changes that occur as the baby is born, the placenta is delivered, and lactation begins. It is also important that the expectant mother discuss her plans to breastfeed with her physician or midwife. The health care provider can work together with the mother to plan the details of delivery and postpartum care to facilitate lactation.

Having made the decision to breastfeed and having prepared herself for it, a woman must learn *how* to nurse her new baby. Included here are chapters that cover methods of increasing milk production and release, or let-down, and what to do when small problems arise. The author also describes more complicated problems, though these are rare, and explains the course of treatment a doctor or midwife is likely to recommend. It is important to recognize when a situation warrants medical attention, since early appropriate management can usually minimize a problem and facilitate its resolution.

The author, who has breastfed her own children, is also a perinatal nurse who has counseled thousands of new mothers through a breast-feeding clinic and telephone hot line. With her practical experience enhanced by her formal study of lactation, she is especially qualified to prepare this manual for mothers.

A new mother needs to be confident that she is doing the best for her baby. This book will give her the knowledge that is vital to developing that confidence. With the rich store of information herein, every mother should be able to experience the joy of breastfeeding.

RUTH A. LAWRENCE, M.D.

*University of Rochester*

# Preface

Not long ago, a first-time nursing mother came to me about a difficulty she was having breastfeeding her baby. After we successfully resolved it, she suggested I write a book on breastfeeding that included problem-solving techniques. Although I was flattered, such a project seemed monumental. But later, as I recalled her enthusiasm, I began to consider the insights I had gained over years of assisting so many mothers, first as a maternity and newborn nurse and later after founding a breastfeeding clinic and telephone counseling service. Certainly, I was more than familiar with the common concerns of mothers who are learning to breastfeed, as well as with the occasional problems that can interfere with the development of a successful nursing relationship. The next day I wrote my rough outline.

Many excellent books had already been written on the benefits of nursing over artificial feeding methods. I set out, however, to provide mothers with a practical guide for easy reference throughout the nursing period. The first part of the book provides basic information about the breast, preparation for nursing, and nursing during the first week; the remainder of the book is intended for reading as the baby and the nursing relationship grow and develop. There are chapters on each of the three later phases of nursing—from the first week through the second month, from the second month through the sixth, and after the sixth month. Following each of these chapters is a Survival Guide—a quick yet thorough reference for almost any problem you or your baby may encounter during the phase covered. Although you may rarely need to consult the Survival Guides, I have included them to ensure that, when you do, you will be able to identify and resolve your problem as quickly as possible. Because many nursing women occasionally find themselves in need of medication, Dr. Philip Anderson has provided an appendix on drugs and their safety for the breast-fed baby.

During the year I spent writing this book, I received a great deal of encouragement and guidance. I am tremendously indebted to Lynn Moen for her support along the way. I also wish to thank Penny Simkin, R.P.T., and my editor, Linda Ziedrich, for their many efforts on my behalf.

For their thoughtful review of the text I thank Marian Tompson; Andrea Herron, R.N., M.S., C.L.C.; Kathleen Rodriquez Michaelson, B.A., C.L.C.; Vicki McDonald, R.D.; Judith La Vigna; Julie Merrill, R.N.; Tom Robinson; and Kathleen Auerbach, Ph.D.

Jim Litzenburger; Vicki Gadberry, R.N., C.N.M.; Marilyn Worth, R.N.; Kathleen Long, M.D.; and Dawn Edwards, R.N.C., are most appreciated for their encouragement as well as their friendship.

I am grateful to Donna Janetski for her commitment to this project in preparing the manuscript. My thanks also to Mike Sims for his generosity, and to Susan and Kirk Graves for their efforts.

This book would never have been possible without my husband, Brad, whose love, patience, and faith sustained me. Kate, my twelve-year-old and former nursing companion, was my inspiration throughout.

NOTE TO THE SECOND EDITION: For assistance in preparing this edition I would like to thank Trina Vosti, I.B.C.L.C., and Andrea VanOutryve, I.B.C.L.C. And thanks to John, my current nursing companion.

*THE* *Nursing*
*Mother's*
*Companion*

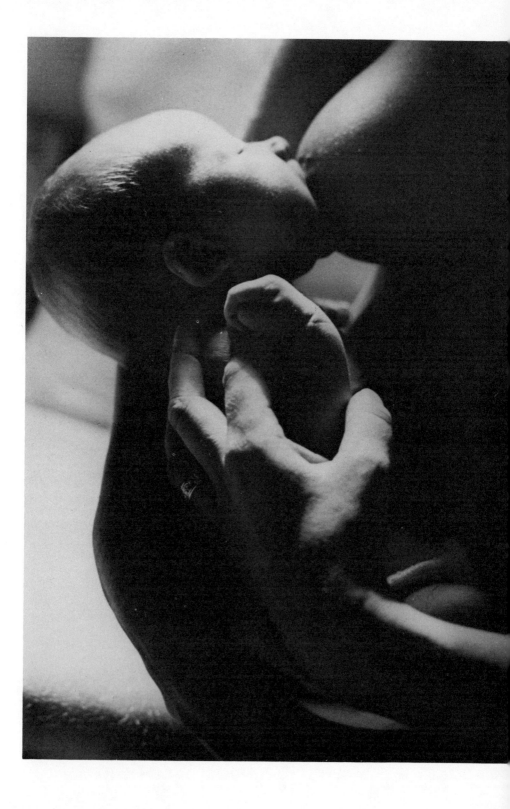

# Introduction

SINCE THE BEGINNING OF HUMANKIND, WOMEN HAVE PUT THEIR IN-
fants to breast. Extending the physical bond that begins at conception,
they have nourished and protected their young with their bodies.
These tender moments, in return, have brought pleasure and fulfill-
ment to the task of mothering. If you are now pregnant, you are probably looking forward to the time in which you will nourish, comfort,
and protect your child in the same way as others before you—at the
breast.

Perhaps you already feel committed to the idea of nursing. For you,
there is no question that you'll breastfeed your baby. Or perhaps, like
many women, you have some uncertainties, but still feel it's worth a
try. Your outlook depends on many things—the value you place on
breastfeeding, how your partner feels about it, how your friends have
fed their babies, your lifestyle, your feelings about yourself and your
body.

You probably also have some notions about what nursing will be
like. Perhaps you think it will be easy and convenient. Maybe you
worry that it might not fit in with your activities and plans. You may
have concerns about your ability to nurse. Probably you know of
other women who tried to nurse but soon gave up. Whatever your
attitudes, expectations, and concerns about breastfeeding, these may
become powerful determinants in your ultimate success or failure to
nurse your baby happily.

## Is Breastfeeding Really Better?

You may be under the impression that the decision to breastfeed or
bottle-feed is simply a matter of personal preference. Don't let anyone
fool you into believing that breast milk and formula are equally
good—they are not. Without a doubt, mother's milk alone promotes
optimum health for babies. It is uniquely designed to meet the complete nutritional needs of the growing human infant. It also protects
the infant against illness throughout the entire first year and beyond,
as long as nursing continues.

Although babies do grow on processed infant formulas, formula
manufacturers are continually challenged to include all of the nutrients in breast milk that scientists are gradually identifying as important components of infant growth and development. But artificial infant milks, whether based on cow milk or soybeans, will never be
able to duplicate nature's formula. Human milk contains proteins that
promote brain development and specific immunities against human
illness. In contrast, cow milk contains proteins that favor muscular

growth and specific immunities to bovine disease. Babies, like all young mammals, do best with milk from their own species. Babies on a formula diet are at greater risk for illness and hospitalization. Diarrheal infections, respiratory illnesses, and ear infections are more frequent and serious among these babies. Formula-fed infants also have higher incidences of colic, constipation, and allergic disorders. In fact, a significant number of babies are allergic to formulas, both those based on cow milk and those based on soy. There is also some evidence that artificially fed infants more often experience learning disorders and lower levels of intellectual functioning (American Academy of Pediatrics, 1984).

Bottle feeding with formula more commonly leads to overfeeding and obesity, which may well persist into childhood, adolescence, and adulthood. Tooth decay, malocclusion (improper meeting of the upper and lower teeth), and distortion of the facial muscles may also directly result from sucking on bottles.

Some studies suggest the benefits of breastfeeding also extend into adulthood. Breastfed babies have lower cholesterol levels, on average, when they become adults. Although asthma rates are not significantly different between breastfed and non-breastfed babies, there is a lower rate of asthma in adults who were breastfed. Babies born into diabetic families have a smaller chance of developing the disease themselves if they are breastfed. For all of these reasons, the American Academy of Pediatrics recommends that infants be offered only breast milk for the first four to six months after birth, and that breastfeeding continue throughout the entire first year.

Establishing a close bond and meeting the emotional needs of a child are certainly an essential part of mothering. The nursing woman is thought to produce hormones that promote a physiologic bonding between mother and child. And in what better way can a baby be nurtured, comforted, and made to feel secure than snuggled within his mother's loving arms, against the warmth of her breast? Although some rationalize that bottle-feeding mothers can capture a similar warm feeding relationship, in reality they do not. This is partly because bottle feeding doesn't require much human contact. The bottle-fed baby generally receives less stroking, caressing, and rocking than the breastfed baby. He is talked to less often and he spends more time in his crib away from his parents. Although it is unknown how prevalent the practice of propping bottles for the young infant is, probably the overwhelming majority of babies who are able hold their own bottles and become almost entirely responsible for feeding themselves.

## Practical Considerations

Although you may already be convinced nursing is best for your baby, you may have heard it will be a bother for you.

Which is more convenient, breast or bottle feeding? Whereas formula-feeding mothers feel they are less "tied down," most experienced nursing mothers are grateful they don't have to shop for formula and prepare bottles. It's difficult to believe that getting up at night to fix a bottle is more convenient than pulling the baby to the breast and dozing off again. Outings with a nursing baby mean not having to cart around formula, bottles, and nipples wherever you go. Just because the breastfed baby is easy to take along doesn't mean she can't be left behind; you can leave milk for your infant at times the two of you must be apart.

Mothers who plan to return to work often worry whether they will be able to continue nursing. Today, a growing number of women are combining motherhood, nursing, and working, and doing it quite successfully. Having a healthy baby is especially important, and breastfed babies are sick less often. And to a working mother, after several hours spent apart, moreover, nursing becomes a loving reunion between a working mother and her child (see Chapter 5).

Expectant mothers often hear stories about women who tried to nurse their babies but failed. Perhaps you know women who claim that they didn't produce enough milk, that it wasn't rich enough, that their milk supply dried up one day, that their milk didn't agree with their baby, or that the baby suddenly decided he wanted a bottle instead. You may even have heard that women with small breasts or those who are "nervous types" aren't able to nurse.

Maybe you put no stock in these common myths, and believe instead that because nursing a baby is natural it must be easy. Sometimes it isn't. Today close to half of all mothers who start out nursing their babies give it up within the first six weeks. The reason for this failure is rarely that the mother is unable to produce enough milk. Typically it is because she is alone in her efforts to nurse. All too many new mothers know little about the nursing process and the breastfed infant, have little or no guidance, and lack support while they are learning. Although breastfeeding is natural, it is not instinctive—it must be learned.

When anticipating nursing, some women worry about modesty. Although we all know making milk is the natural function of our breasts, most of us feel embarrassed about exposing them. At first you may be more comfortable nursing in private, but most women find that with a little time and experience, nursing in the presence of others can be discreet and comfortable. Techniques for discreet nursing are discussed in Chapter 5.

You may have heard that nursing can be painful. Normally, women find it comfortable and pleasurable. Some women worry about developing sore nipples during the early days of nursing, but most soreness can be avoided by correctly positioning the baby at the breast (see Chapter 2). You may have also heard that babies sometimes bite their mothers while nursing. When a baby is sucking his tongue covers his lower gums and teeth so he cannot bite. Still, some babies do occasionally bite at the end of feeding, usually during a period of teething. Most babies learn very quickly not to do this.

Pregnancy typically causes the breasts to enlarge, and sometimes to develop stretch marks. During the first few months of nursing, women whose breasts are normally small or medium-sized generally find them to be bigger. Women whose breasts are normally large can usually expect them to stay about the same size as they were late in pregnancy. As the baby gets older and begins nursing less often, most women notice their breasts reduce in size. At weaning, the breasts typically appear smaller still and somewhat droopy, but within six months they generally resume their usual size and shape. Whether you nurse or not, however, you may notice a change in the firmness of your breasts after you have a baby. Childbearing, not nursing, is along with age and heredity a major determinant of the breasts' ultimate appearance.

## What's in It for Mom?

Although the health of an infant and the emotional benefits of breastfeeding are certainly reason enough to nurse, mothers frequently have other motives.

Experienced nursing mothers boast about the ease and convenience of breastfeeding. They are often quick to add that information, guidance, support, and reassurance were essential at the start. After the first few weeks, however, nursing a baby simplifies life considerably.

Many women worry about how they will look after they have had a baby. The fat you accumulate during pregnancy is intended for caloric reserves while nursing. Although vigorous dieting is not a good idea during the nursing period, most mothers find that they gradually lose weight while they are breastfeeding, so long as they are not overeating.

Many studies report lower breast cancer rates among women who have breastfed, and it appears that the risk of cancer decreases the longer a woman nurses. There is some evidence, too, that nursing offers protection against osteoporosis (brittle bones), which can occur later in life. And breastfeeding generally lengthens the time before menstrual periods resume. Most nursing women find they don't have a menstrual cycle for several months after delivery, so long as they are nursing frequently.

All nursing mothers appreciate the money they save by not buying formula. Mothers committed to providing their children with wholesome, natural foods see breast milk as a sound beginning. Some mothers are frankly offended by the smell and taste of many formula preparations, not to mention the unpleasant odor of the bowel movements and spit up milk of the formula-fed baby, and the stains formula may leave on clothing.

Mothers who nurse do so not only because they want the very best nourishment and protection for their babies and because they personally derive many practical benefits from breastfeeding, but simply because they enjoy the experience. The loving relationship established between mother and infant at the breast is emotionally fulfilling and pleasurable. You'll know no greater reward as a mother than witnessing your child grow from your body—first in the womb, and then at the breast.

*Photo essay by Harriette Hartigan*

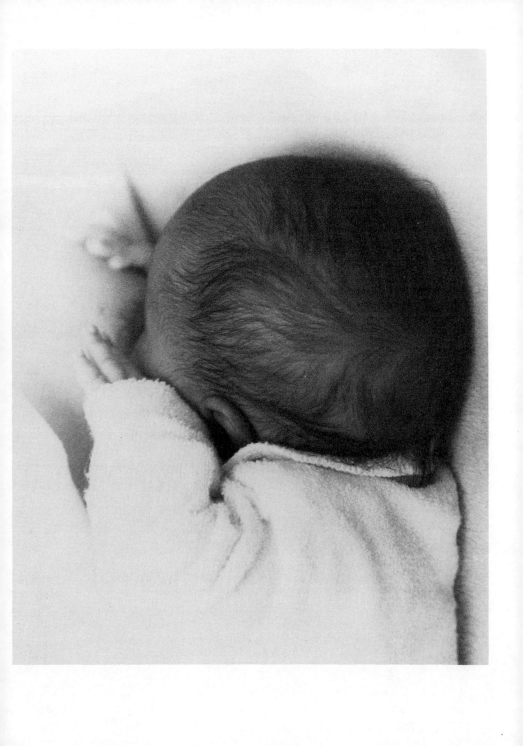

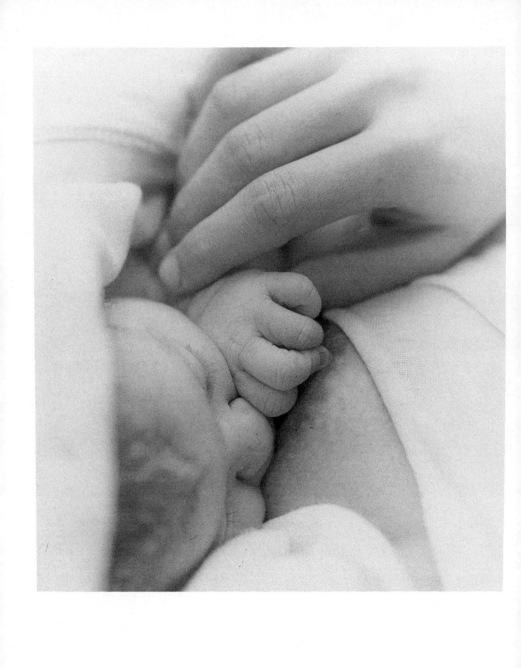

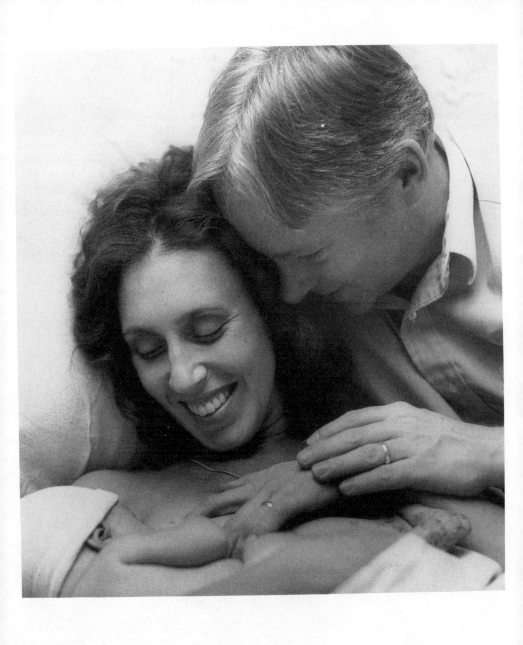

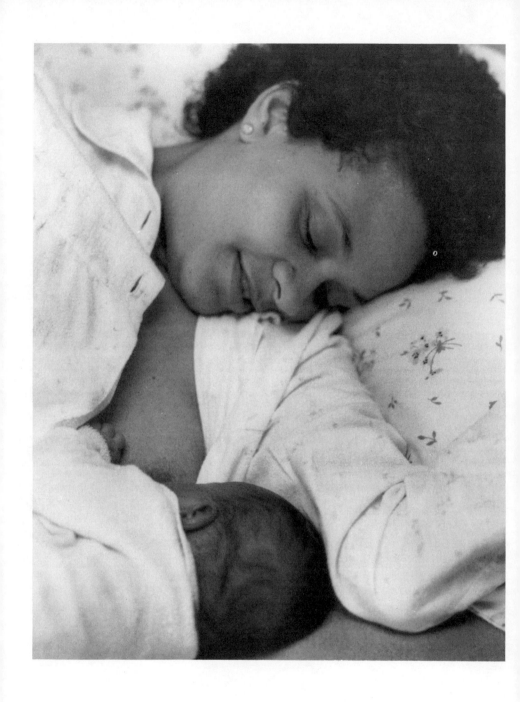

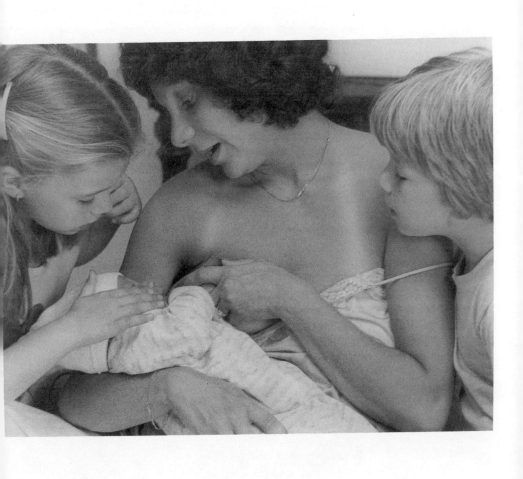

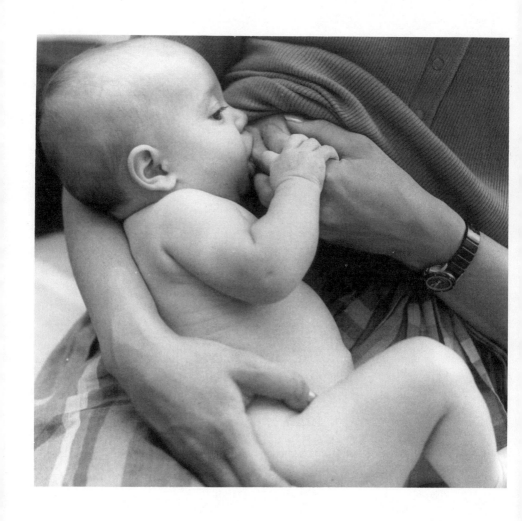

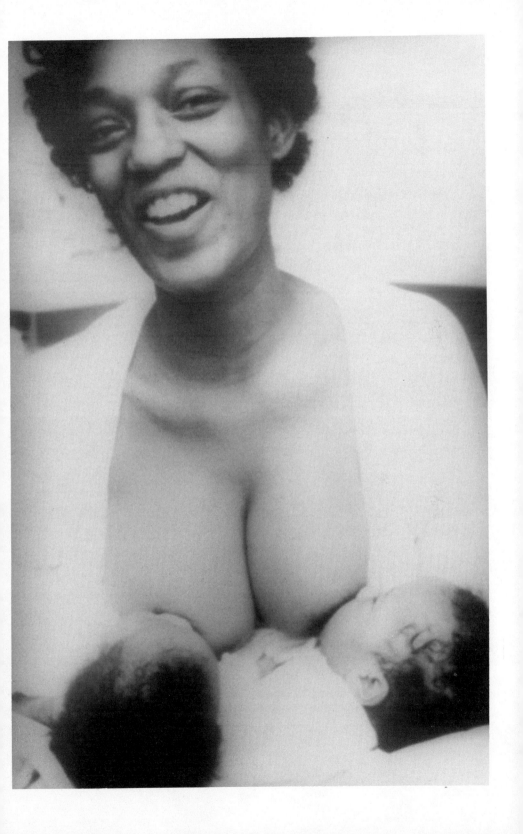

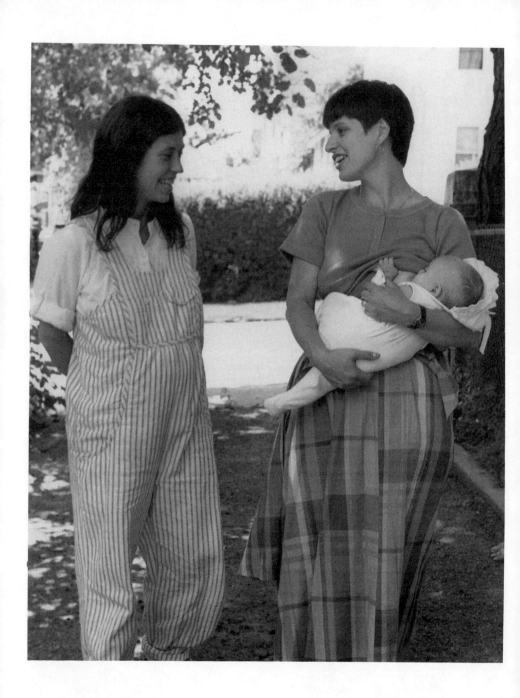

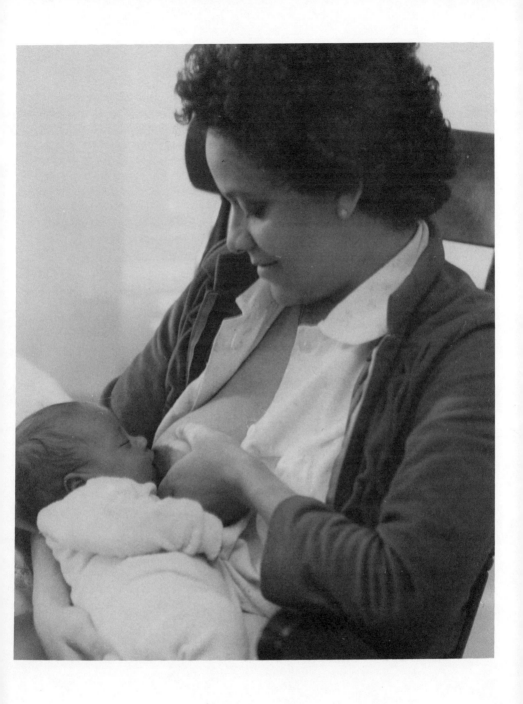

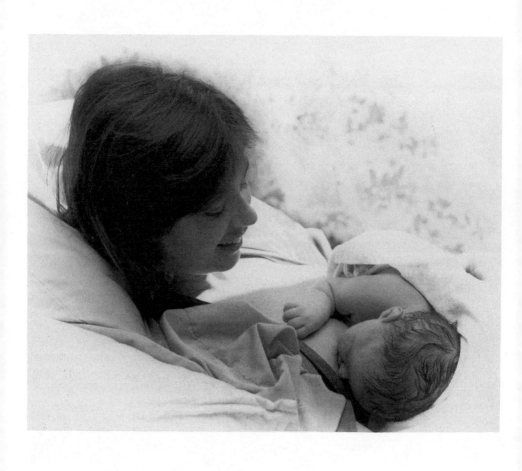

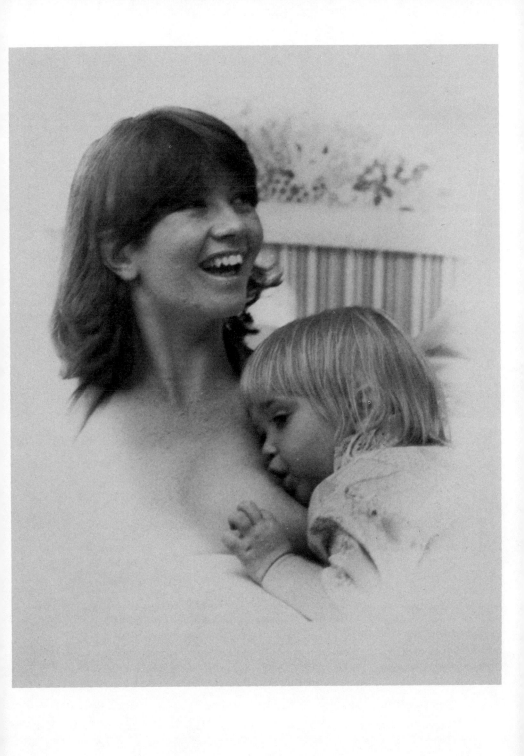

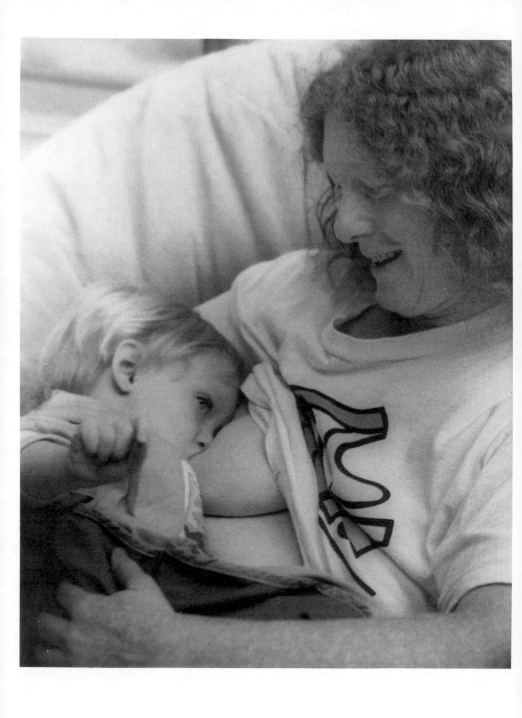

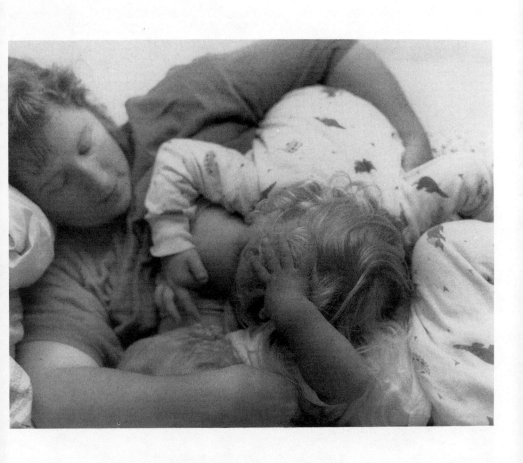

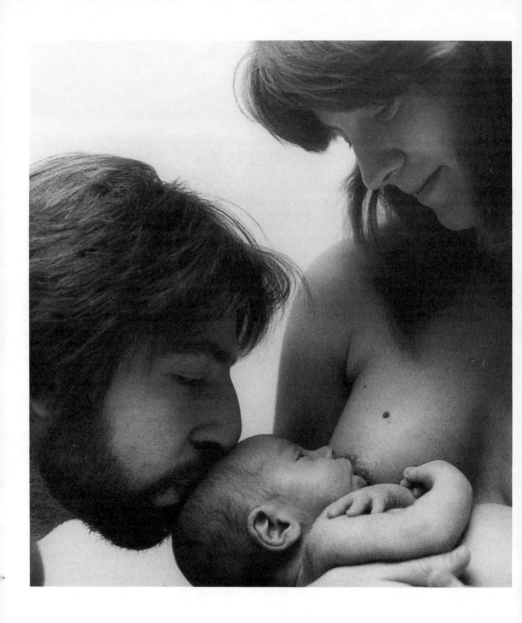

*Sweet voice, sweet lips, soft hands, and softer breast.*

JOHN KEATS

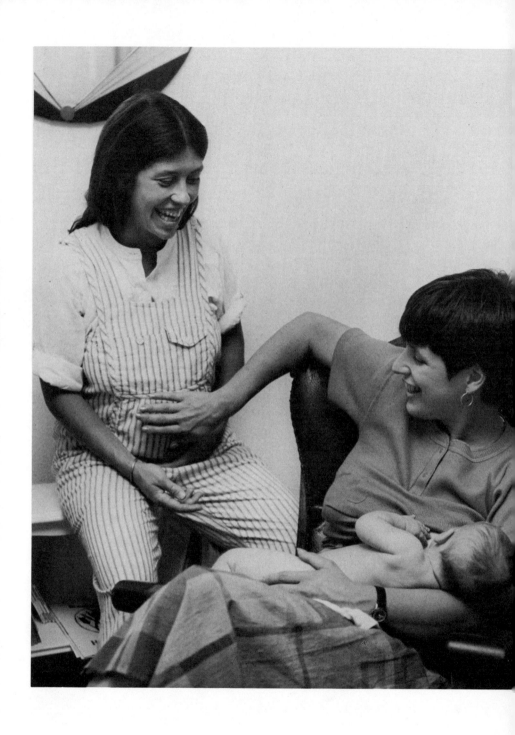

# *Looking Forward: Preparations during Pregnancy*

YOU MAY HAVE DECIDED TO NURSE YOUR BABY LONG BEFORE YOU became pregnant. Or perhaps you have just begin to consider breast-feeding. Although nourishing a baby at the breast is natural, many new mothers are surprised to find it is a learned skill—one that usually takes several weeks to master.

Success at nursing often depends upon a woman's confidence and commitment. You can develop your confidence by learning as much as possible about breastfeeding ahead of time. You can strengthen your commitment to nurse by developing a strong support system for yourself.

## Learning about Breastfeeding

Generations ago, most new mothers turned to their own mothers for support and guidance on breastfeeding. Unfortunately, few women today can do this. For many, the art of breastfeeding is learned alone—by trial and error. All too often this leads to frustration and discouragement.

There are several ways you can learn about nursing ahead of time. Reading about it is certainly beneficial. In some communities breast-feeding classes are offered. Expectant mothers are also most welcome to attend La Leche League meetings, which are held monthly in most areas. La Leche League is the organization of nursing mothers whose purpose is to support breastfeeding worldwide. In some areas, other groups such as the Nursing Mothers Counsel provide classes and tele-phone counseling for pregnant and nursing women. These groups are listed in Appendix A. In addition, hospitals, county health depart-ments, and WIC (Women, Infants, and Children) programs may spon-sor prenatal breastfeeding classes.

Another excellent way to learn about breastfeeding is to spend time with women who are nursing their babies. It may be that you have never seen, close up, a mother and baby breastfeeding. Most nursing mothers will delight in your interest, and one or two may become good sources of information and support for you in the days to come. Be sure to ask them about their first weeks of nursing. Most likely you will hear of a variety of experiences, and perhaps you will develop a sense of what the early period of breastfeeding can be like.

## Your Breasts

During pregnancy many changes occur in your breasts in preparation for nourishing your baby. Initially, you probably noticed they were more full and tender than usual. Their increasing size during the first

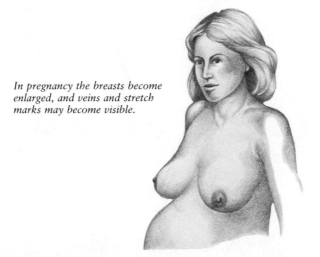

*In pregnancy the breasts become enlarged, and veins and stretch marks may become visible.*

few months of pregnancy is caused by the development of the milk-making structures within them. With this growth the blood flow to the breasts increases, and veins in the breasts may become clearly visible. Some women develop stretch marks on their breasts like the ones that can occur on the abdomen during pregnancy.

The nipple and the area around the nipple, the areola, double in size and deepen in color; this darkening may serve as a visual cue to the newborn. Also during this time, small glands located in the areola, known as Montgomery's tubercles, become pronounced. Their function is to secrete an antibacterial lubricant that keeps the nipple moist and protected during pregnancy and breastfeeding. This is why soaps and special creams are unnecessary in caring for your breasts, and may even be harmful: soaps remove the breast's natural lubricant, and creams may interfere with its antibacterial action.

The nipples often become more sensitive during pregnancy in preparation for nursing. Some women may find that their nipples are overly sensitive and even hurt when touched. Other women enjoy this sensitivity and feel great pleasure when their breasts are fondled during lovemaking.

By the fifth or sixth month of pregnancy, the breasts are fully capable of producing milk. Some women begin to notice drops of fluid on the nipple at this time. This fluid, known as colostrum, comes from the many tiny openings in the nipple and is the food your baby will receive during the first few days after birth. Some women do not leak colostrum, but it is there in the breasts just the same.

As women, we all receive messages about our bodies and what they

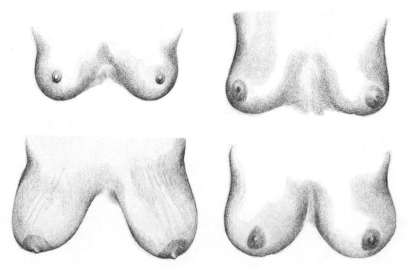

*Breasts come in all sizes and shapes.*

"ought" to look like. These messages affect our self-image, including our feelings about our breasts and how they look. You can probably remember how you felt about your breasts as they developed in early adolescence. You may have felt proud as they grew larger and you began wearing a bra. Perhaps you were embarrassed if they developed earlier or grew larger than the other girls'. You may have felt anxious if they took a long time to grow, or self-conscious if they were small.

Even now you may wish that your breasts were smaller or larger, fuller or less droopy. You may not resemble the women with "perfect" breasts portrayed in photographs of nursing mothers. Hopefully, though, you accept your breasts and feel good about them regardless of their size or shape.

Each woman's breasts are very different from all others, but the breast, regardless of size, is perfectly designed for its ultimate purpose—to nourish and nurture our children. The breasts not only provide an infant with superb nutrients for growth and development, but offer the warmth, the love, and the security that every growing baby needs. In this respect, they are most beautiful.

**Caring for your breasts.** During the last months of pregnancy, rinse your breasts in your bath or shower. Avoid soaping them, since soaps tend to dry the nipples and the areola. If your breasts are dry or itchy, a mild cream or lotion may feel soothing, but avoid getting it on the nipple or areola.

Many women prefer to wear a supportive bra during pregnancy, although some are just as comfortable without one.

**The making and giving of milk.** After the birth of your baby, colostrum is readily available for her first nursings. Colostrum is the ideal food for her first days; it is both perfect nutritionally and important for protection against infection. Milk generally appears by the second or third day, but occasionally not until the fourth or fifth.

Your body is signaled to initiate milk production with the delivery of the placenta. This causes the hormone prolactin to activate the milk-producing cells of the breast. The initial manufacture of milk occurs whether the baby nurses or not; it can be prevented only by taking a medication for the purpose soon after delivery. Continued milk production is another matter. This depends on frequent and reg-

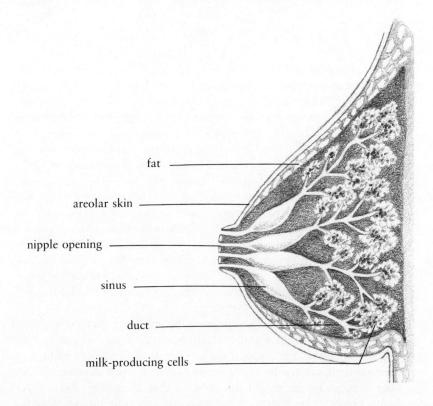

fat

areolar skin

nipple opening

sinus

duct

milk-producing cells

*Cross-section of a lactating breast.*

ular stimulation of the breast and the release of milk. The baby's sucking stimulates the nerve endings in the breast, which in turn trigger
the release of the two hormones essential to milk production and release—prolactin and oxytocin.

Prolactin, as mentioned previously, activates the milk-producing
cells in the breast to manufacture milk. Oxytocin is responsible for
the release of the milk from the tiny sacs where the milk is made. This
release is referred to as the ejection or let-down reflex. As the baby
nurses, the milk is propelled forward to the sinuses beneath the areola.
It is the baby's job to get the milk out of the sinuses by compressing
the areola with her tongue and gums as she nurses.

During the early months of her life, your baby will receive plenty
of milk as long as she nurses frequently, at least eight times in 24
hours, is sucking properly, and is allowed a sufficient amount of time
to complete each feeding. This is because breastfeeding works by supply and demand. The more your breasts are stimulated by the baby's
sucking, the more milk you will produce.

## Planning for the First Days

**Nipple preparation.** Often mothers who plan to breastfeed are advised
to prepare their nipples during pregnancy. In fact, studies have shown
that nipple "toughening" maneuvers such as brisk rubbing or twisting
do little to prevent soreness during early breastfeeding. Whether or
not they have especially sensitive skin, blondes and redheads do not
generally experience any more nipple soreness than other women.
Sore nipples are usually prevented by correctly positioning the baby
at the breast during nursing (see Chapter 2).

Some women are also instructed to express colostrum every day
during the last six weeks of pregnancy to prevent engorgement, or
swelling of the breasts, when milk production begins. Again, there is
no evidence that expressing colostrum has any beneficial effect on
later engorgement. Many specialists discourage this practice because
it may stimulate uterine contractions and, possibly, premature labor.
Little is known about other possible effects of the intentional removal
of this valuable fluid.

One preparation is very important during pregnancy: you should
make sure your nipples can extend outward. Your baby may have
difficulty grasping the breast if the nipples do not protrude enough on
their own or cannot be made to protrude. Do not assume because
your nipples appear to extend outward that all is well. Even if you
had a breast exam earlier in your pregnancy, your nipples may not

| Normal nipple appearance | Appearance when pinched | |
|---|---|---|
| | *Satisfactory* | *Needs correction* |
| Protruding | Nipple stays protruded | Nipple moves inward or flattens |
| Flat | Nipple can be pinched outward | Nipple moves inward or cannot be pinched outward |
| Dimpled or folded | Entire nipple extends outward | Nipple moves inward or flattens |
| Inverted | Entire nipple extends outward | Nipple extends out only slightly, remains inverted, or inverts further |

have been fully checked. Take the time to perform your own assessment.

First, look at both your nipples. They may protrude, or one or both may be flat, dimpled, folded in the center, or inverted. Next, do the "pinch test": gently squeeze just behind the nipple with your thumb and forefinger. This imitates the motion your baby will make while nursing. See how both nipples respond. If your nipples are flat, pull them outward to determine if they can lift away from the inner mass of the breast. The following chart will help you determine whether you need to take further steps to minimize initial nursing difficulties.

*When nipples need correction.* The flat nipple that cannot be pinched outward, or the nipple that moves inward or flattens when compressed, is said to be "tied" to the inner breast tissue by tiny adhe-

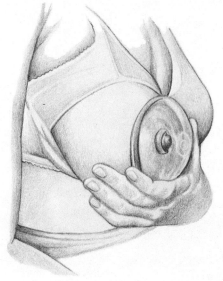

*Breast shells can improve nipple shape.*

sions. The physical changes of pregnancy help the nipples to stand out, but one or both may still need correction. In this case, special plastic breast shells may solve the problem before breastfeeding begins.

Worn inside the bra, breast shells exert a steady but gentle pressure on the areola and cause the nipple to extend outward through the opening in the shell. This helps to loosen the adhesions beneath the nipple. Breast shells should be worn as soon as you have determined that improvement is needed, ideally from about mid-pregnancy on. They can be purchased in most maternity shops (see Appendix A for information on ordering them). Gradually work up to wearing the shells most of the day, letting comfort be your guide.

**The postpartum setting.** Too few mothers realize ahead of time the tremendous effect the immediate postpartum experience—in a hospital, in a birth center, or at home—can have on their breastfeeding success. It is most worthwhile to evaluate the situation you will be in after delivery to make any necessary arrangements for early nursing.

Some women have the opportunity to select among several hospitals or birth centers for their delivery. If you are making such a choice, be sure to get a recommendation from your childbirth educator or a breastfeeding counselor. She will probably know which places are most supportive of nursing mothers and infants. Even if only one hospital is available to you—and many birth attendants practice at only one—it is well worth your time to ask about the policies of the maternity unit. This will help assure that your nursing gets off to the best possible start.

Take advantage of the maternity tours, teas, and classes that most hospitals and birth centers offer, or call the postpartum unit (make sure the nurse has time to talk) to learn about policies and routines. Be sure to inquire:

- How soon after delivery will I be able to nurse? What if I have a cesarean birth?
- How often is nursing encouraged during the day and at night?
- Can the baby stay in the room with me? If not, how often and for how long will we be together?
- What assistance with breastfeeding is offered by the nursing staff?
- Does the staff avoid supplemental bottle feeding?
- Is there a lactation professional on staff?

If the nurse is friendly and receptive to your questions, you might also ask which pediatricians she feels are particularly knowledgeable about breastfeeding and supportive of it.

Ideally, the maternity unit's policies encourage mothers and babies to remain together for the first few hours after birth, or at least assure that nursing takes place within the first two hours, when the baby is likely to be alert and eager to suck. Breastfeeding goes best when nursing is frequent, every one to three hours, during both day and night. "Rooming in" with the baby, at least during the day and evening, is conducive to frequent nursing and allows the mother and baby to become better acquainted before going home. Preferably, the nursing staff does not routinely give the babies water or formula supplements, as this lessens their interest in nursing and sometimes interferes with their ability to breastfeed. It can be an added bonus if the nurses enjoy assisting breastfeeding mothers or if one nurse is specifically responsible for breastfeeding counseling.

If you are planning an early discharge from a hospital or birth center, or will be delivering at home, you may also want to inquire about home visits by a nurse or midwife during the first few days.

**The baby's doctor.** Your breastfeeding experience can be greatly influenced by your choice of physician for your child. You may want a pediatrician for your baby, or you may prefer to use a family practitioner (you may certainly choose to continue with a family practitioner who attended your baby's birth). In selecting a doctor, start by getting the names of those who are known to have a positive attitude about breastfeeding. Ask your obstetrician, midwife, childbirth educator, or a lactation professional for recommendations. You might also inquire about physicians in your area who work with nurse practitioners. These nurses have advanced education and training in well-baby care, and they usually provide mothers with extra attention and counseling on a variety of parental concerns, including breastfeeding.

Most doctors and nurse practitioners will set aside time for a preliminary visit with expectant parents. Sometimes this is free of charge; they realize you are "looking and choosing." Be sure to visit at least two before making a final decision, even if the first one seems nice. By all means meet the office nurse. She will often be the one who will answer your questions or concerns when you call during office hours. She can be a good resource for you, especially if she has breastfed successfully herself or has a special interest in nursing.

Let the doctor or nurse practitioner know that you are going to nurse your baby. Ask what proportion of the babies in the practice are breastfed; the answer will give you a clue to his or her overall support of nursing mothers. Take time to discuss your preferences for feeding the baby in the hospital. If the maternity unit's policies are not ideal, ask for written orders to allow early nursing and rooming-in, and to prevent the feeding of supplements to your baby.

There may be other questions you will want to ask about the hospital or birth center, or about well-baby care. Bring a list with you so you don't forget any of them. Be sure to inquire about any necessary procedures for notifying the doctor or nurse practitioner when the baby is born. It is often said that the pediatrician takes care of the parents perhaps even more than the child. Trust your intuition when making your final choice about which pediatrician, family doctor, or nurse practitioner is right for you.

**Nursing bras and pads.** Though nursing bras are not an absolute necessity, most mothers find them convenient during the early weeks of breastfeeding. The ideal features of a nursing bra include nonelastic straps for sufficient support, front flap fasteners that are manageable with one hand, and plastic-free cotton cups that permit air circulation to the nipples.

It is important to select a bra that fits properly. Shop for your bras about two weeks before your due date; at this time your breasts will be close to the size they will be during early nursing. When trying bras on, fasten them on the outside row of hooks, as your rib cage will probably decrease in size after delivery. Choose a cup size that supports the underside of the breast comfortably. The upper side of the cup should be looser or expandable so that there there will be room for the breast to grow when milk production begins, and for a breast pad or shell. Evaluate underwire bras cautiously; they can lead to

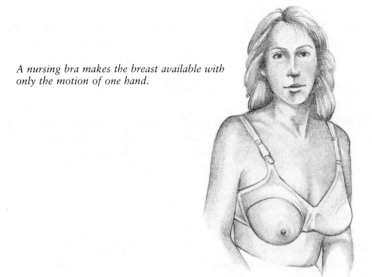

*A nursing bra makes the breast available with
only the motion of one hand.*

plugged milk ducts and breast infections if the wires press into the
side of the breast or limit blood circulation. Stretch bras that can be
pulled out of the way may work just as well for you as nursing bras
if you are small-breasted.

The salesperson in the maternity shop or department may be very
helpful when you are making your selection. To be on the safe side,
it is probably best to limit your purchase to two bras. After a week or
so of nursing, you will be more sure of the size and style you are most
comfortable with.

You may wish to purchase breast pads before delivery, to keep your
bra and clothing dry during the early weeks of nursing. These pads
come in two varieties, disposable and reusable. Whichever you select,
be sure the pads do not contain plastic or waterproof liners, as these
can contribute to nipple soreness. (Not all women leak, so you may
want to start with just one pack.) Some women prefer to use handker-
chiefs or cut-up cloth diapers instead of commercial pads.

Sometimes mothers consider using plastic breast shells instead of
pads to keep dry. The primary purpose of these shells is to improve
nipple shape. When they are routinely worn in place of pads, milk
may leak excessively.

**Other purchases you may be considering.** The arms of an adult are
never a safe place for an infant or small child riding in an automobile.

If you use a car, you should purchase an infant restraining seat; depending on the state you live in, you may be legally required to use it. You may wish to check with your baby's doctor or automobile association for a listing of car seats that are approved by safety experts. These seats can be quite expensive, so you will want to compare prices carefully. Some communities and hospitals offer car seat rental and loan programs.

Many mothers enjoy using infant carriers. These soft "pouches" or slings are a comfortable and convenient way to carry the baby with your arms free for other things. Most babies are quite happy to be snuggled next to their mother's or father's body in one of these.

Besides being ecologically safer than disposable diapers, cloth diapers are more economical as well, if you own or have access to a washer and dryer.

You may want to arrange for diaper service for the first few weeks. Full service is usually no more expensive than disposable diapers and is a luxury all new parents deserve.

Some mothers buy breast pumps before delivery. Although a pump is not a necessity, you may at some time want to use one. Or you may prefer to learn the technique of manual expression, which is described in Chapter 5. If you do decide to purchase a pump ahead of time, see Chapter 5 for a review of the more popular types.

## Planning for the First Weeks

During your first few weeks of motherhood, caring for the baby and yourself will take just about all of your time and energy. Most new mothers find they are often tired and have emotional highs and lows. Planning ahead can make these important first weeks go much more smoothly for both you and your family.

If your partner can possibly manage to take time off from work, by all means encourage him to do so. Not only can he help in fixing meals, managing the household, and caring for any other children at home, but he also needs and deserves time to get to know the baby. And he can be a great source of support and encouragement while you are learning to breastfeed.

Other family members can also make these weeks easier, but invite them to stay with you only if you feel they will make a positive contribution and be supportive of your nursing.

Perhaps some of your friends in the area have already offered to help when the baby arrives. There are many things they can do, like fixing a meal, washing a load or two of laundry, running errands, minding any older children, or spending an hour or so straightening up your house.

It's also a good idea to stock up on groceries before the birth. Include foods that are easy to prepare and plenty of things to drink. You may also want to plan some simple menus or freeze some dinners ahead of time.

**Your support system.** About half of American women who start out breastfeeding give up and begin bottle feeding within the first two months after birth. As said so well by Dana Raphael (1976), "The odds in our culture today are stacked heavily against successful breastfeeding, and the emotional price for failure is high." Mothers frequently give up breastfeeding in the learning stage because they have little information, guidance, and support.

When a nursing mother is encouraged and cared for by others, her motivation can carry her through almost any difficult situation. When she feels alone and unsupported, however, the nursing relationship seems to fall apart at the slightest provocation.

As enthusiastic as you feel now, you probably have difficulty imagining that during the early weeks you may sometimes doubt your ability to nurse. In fact, many new mothers experience periods of anxiety while they are learning to breastfeed. If you are lucky you can turn to your own mother for advice and reassurance about nursing. Many of our mothers, however, nursed us only a few weeks, if at all. You may hear from today's grandmothers that "no one nursed back then," "the doctor said the bottle was easier," "I just didn't make enough milk," or "the doctor said my milk wasn't rich enough." Comments such as these reflect an era when women received little encouragement and support in their efforts to nurse, especially from their male doctors. Consider for a moment the idea of giving birth all alone. Awful, right? It is probably important to you that someone you love and trust will be with you, encouraging you each step of the way. During your early weeks of breastfeeding you need the same kind of support—the presence of someone who provides reassurance, guidance, and encouragement.

You may be fortunate enough to have friends who have nursed—or are nursing—their babies, and a partner who believes with you that breastfeeding is healthy and natural. Even so, you may discover in time that not everyone in your life shares your feelings about breastfeeding. If fact, many people feel indifferent, and some downright opposed, to this way of feeding and nurturing a baby. Your partner, mother, or best friend may not be entirely enthusiastic about your decision. Some people may even try to discourage you along the way. Perhaps they feel a bit threatened, fearful, or even jealous of the intimate relationship you will be establishing with the baby. The sad fact of the matter is that despite the renewed enthusiasm of young women today toward breastfeeding, many new mothers still get too little support—from family, friends, health professionals, and society in general.

Develop a support system for yourself ahead of time. Let your partner and other family members know how much breastfeeding means to you and how important they will be to your success. If they have concerns or fears about nursing, find out what they are and provide them with the information they need to correct any misconceptions. If you have older children, talk with them about nursing so they know what to expect. Be sure to identify sources of guidance. Perhaps you are close to women who have successfully nursed their babies. Take time to find the names of lactation professionals in your community. (Your childbirth educator, your maternity unit, or your obstetrician's or pediatrician's nurses may know of some. Two breast pump companies, Medela and Egnell, have geographically-arranged lists of lactation professionals. The companies' toll-free numbers are listed in Appendix A.) When you have gathered these supports, you will have stacked the odds in your favor.

CHAPTER TWO

# Off to a Good Start: The First Week

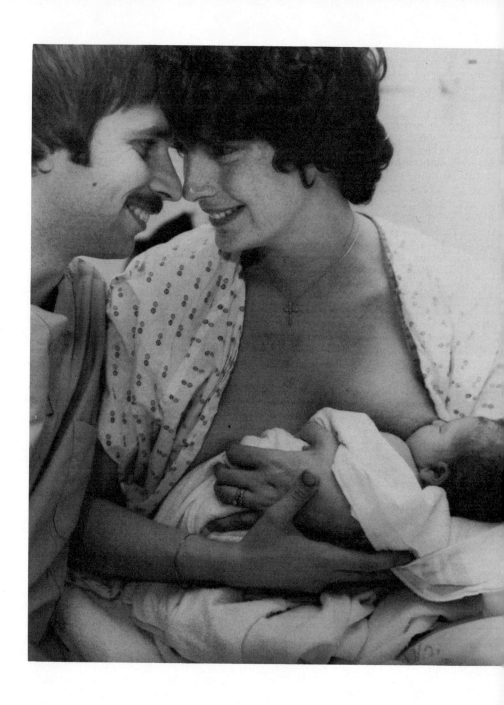

YOU MIGHT EXPECT THAT AFTER THE WORK OF LABOR AND BIRTH A mother and her newborn infant would be too exhausted to greet each other. But no matter how fatigued birth may have left her, the mother usually brightens with renewed energy to explore her baby. Some mothers seem to meet their infants for the first time with puzzlement, as if searching for some sign of familiarity. Others react as if they have always known this tiny being and are overjoyed to meet him at long last.

After several minutes of adjustment to breathing, the temperature change, and lights and sounds, the infant likewise becomes alert, opening his eyes and moving his mouth. Soon he is actively rooting about. With his fists to his mouth, or perhaps his lips against the blanket or his father's arm, he seeks out the comfort of the breast.

## In the Beginning

Throughout the first two hours after birth, the infant is usually alert and eager to suck. At this time he is most ready for his first nursing.

**Colostrum.** It is not unusual to hear a first-time mother tell a nurse, "I don't think I have anything yet to feed the baby." Although small in amount, colostrum is available in the breast in quantities close to the stomach capacity of the newborn. This "liquid gold," which is often yellow but may be clear, resembles blood more than milk in that it contains protective white blood cells capable of attacking harmful bacteria. Colostrum also acts to "seal" the inside of the baby's intestines, preventing the invasion of bacteria, and provides the baby with high levels of antibodies from the mother. Not only does colostrum thus offer protection from sickness, but it is the ideal food for the newborn's first few days of life. It is high in protein and low in sugar and fat, making it easy to digest. Colostrum is also beneficial in stimulating the baby's first bowel movement. The black, tarry stool, called meconium, contains bilirubin, the substance that causes newborn jaundice. Colostrum in frequent doses helps eliminate bilirubin from the body and may lessen the incidence and severity of jaundice.

In the hospital this first nursing may take place in the delivery room, the birthing room, or the recovery area. With minimal assistance from your nurse or partner, the baby will probably latch on eagerly to the breast and suck. He will be more willing if he is unbundled; snuggled within your arm and next to your body, he is unlikely to get too cold (unless perhaps the room is air-conditioned). The purple color of his hands and feet is normal; it is caused by changes in blood circulation that take place at delivery. If you or the nurse is concerned about the cold, place a blanket over the baby after he has begun to nurse.

Many specialists believe that when the first nursing is delayed much beyond the first two hours, the infant may be somewhat reluctant to take the breast thereafter. Nursing without delay also boosts the confidence of the mother, and stimulates the action of hormones that cause the uterus to contract and remain firm after delivery. These contractions may help speed delivery of the placenta and minimize blood loss afterward (breastfeeding alone is insufficient, however, in the case of postpartum hemorrhage, when prompt intervention by the medical staff is essential). During the first few days after birth, some mothers feel these contractions, or "afterpains," while nursing. Mothers who have had other children may be especially uncomfortable with afterpains.

Should you not have the opportunity to nurse right after delivery, or if you can't persuade your baby to take the breast, don't get discouraged. Many mothers have established successful nursing hours or days after giving birth.

**Just the breast.** When you have finished your first nursing in the hospital, let the nurses know (if you have not done so previously) that you prefer your baby be given no supplementary bottles of water or formula and no pacifiers. Water or formula is unnecessary and may confuse your baby while she is learning to breastfeed.

Newborns do not normally require any fluids other than colostrum (the exception is the baby who has low blood sugar—because her mother is diabetic, her birth weight was low, or she underwent unusual stress during labor or delivery). Supplemental feedings, moreover, can be harmful: they may cause the baby to lose interest in the breast and to nurse less frequently than needed. This is because bottle nipples may (1) lessen the baby's instinctive efforts to open her mouth wide, (2) condition her to wait to suck until she feels the firm bottle nipple in her mouth, and (3) encourage her to push her tongue forward—the opposite of what she needs to do while nursing. The baby who has sucked on bottle nipples may also become frustrated while nursing, since milk does not flow as rapidly from the breast as it does from the bottle.

Some hospitals now have policies against giving bottles to nursing newborns, but not all do. To be sure all the nurses know of your preference, ask them to place a sign on the baby's crib like this one:

**To all my nurses:**

While I'm here and learning to breastfeed, PLEASE, NO BOTTLES OR PACIFIERS. My mom will be happy to nurse me whenever I fuss.

Thanks!!
Baby Reynolds

**Time at the breast.** Many doctors and nurses tell mothers that to prevent sore nipples they should limit their nursing time during the first several days. Probably nothing else about breastfeeding is as poorly understood as the causes of sore nipples. It may be explained that keeping feedings short will prevent soreness and will help "toughen" the nipples. Actually, sore nipples usually result from improper positioning of the baby on the breast, not from long nursings. Another myth often heard by new mothers is that the breast "empties" in a prescribed number of minutes. Most newborns require 20 to 40 minutes to complete a feeding. As long as your positioning is correct and nursing is comfortable, there is no need to restrict your nursing time. Besides being unnecessary, limiting nursing time may frustrate the baby and lead to increased engorgement when milk production begins.

**Positioning at the breast.** A baby is correctly positioned at the breast when his gums are on top of the areola, the dark area around the nipples. In this position he will compress the sinuses located beneath

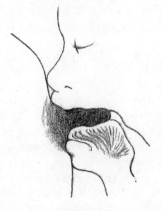

*An infant correctly positioned while nursing.*

the areola to draw out milk. If he instead latches on only to the nipple and starts "chewing," the nipple will probably become sore and cracked, and perhaps even bleed. The baby will also be unable to compress the sinuses beneath the areola and may therefore get too little milk.

Soreness and blisters may also develop when the nipple enters the baby's mouth at an upward angle. This causes the nipple to rub against the roof of the baby's mouth.

Probably the most important skill for you to master, initially, is that of getting the baby on the breast correctly. Some mothers can do this easily, but many need practice. It helps to unwrap the baby first. This will encourage his interest in latching on and make it easier for you to check his position.

*Cuddle hold.* Take time to position yourself comfortably. If you are nursing in a hospital bed, sit as straight as possible with a pillow behind you, or sit on the edge of the bed. Cradle the baby in your arm, his tummy against yours and his head resting in the bend of your elbow, so that he is facing your breast. His lower arm will thus be tucked out of the way, his mouth close to your breast. Your forearm should support the baby's back; your hand should hold his thigh or bottom; and his mouth should be at the level of your nipple (a pillow on your lap may help support him). Support your breast with your free hand; your forearm should cross your body under the unused breast and the upper arm should be relaxed at your side. Place the palm of your hand on your rib cage below the breast, your thumb on top of the breast. Lift the breast so its weight is supported with the palm of your hand. All your fingers should be well behind the areola.

You are now ready to proceed. Your goal is first to stimulate the baby to "root," and then to pull him onto the breast.

- To stimulate the rooting reflex, lightly touch your nipple to the baby's lower lip; he will probably respond by opening his mouth wide.
- As soon as he does, lift your breast upward so the nipple points straight ahead or downward.
- Pull the baby in very close with the arm that holds him, so close that his nose and chin touch the breast. Since he will probably keep his mouth open for only a few seconds, you will need to pull him in quick. Do not lean toward the baby.
- Repeat these steps as many times as necessary until the baby latches on correctly.

Don't worry that the baby won't be able to breathe, though his nose may bury into your breast. After he has taken his first few sucks, you

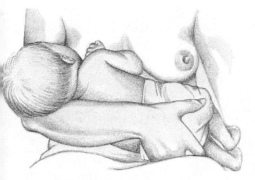

Sit with the baby tummy to tummy.

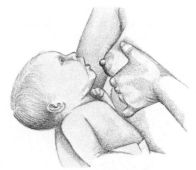

Hold the breast near his mouth.

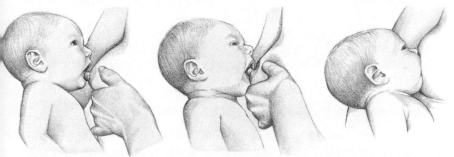

Touch the nipple to his lower lip.        When he opens wide, pull him in to latch on.

can relax the arm you are holding him with, pull his lower trunk and legs closer to you, and, if necessary, depress the top of the breast with your thumb. Once the baby is actively nursing, you may be able to let go of your breast, unless it is too heavy for him to control.

*Cross-cuddle hold.* This hold offers you excellent control over the baby's head when you are pulling him into the breast. As in the cuddle hold, position the baby tummy to tummy, but hold him with the *opposite* arm, so that your hand supports the back of his head. Hold the breast with your free hand. When the baby opens his mouth, you can firmly pull in his head for nursing. After he has latched on, you may want to switch your arms back to the cuddle hold.

*Side-lying position.* The side-lying position is an especially good choice for nursing when—

- You must be flat after a cesarean birth.
- You are uncomfortable sitting up.

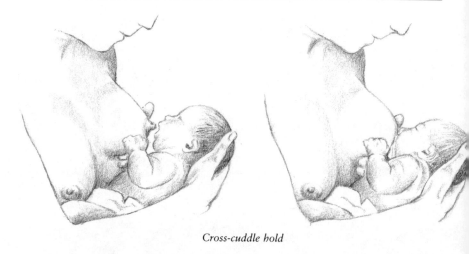

*Cross-cuddle hold*

- You need help from someone else to get the baby latched on.
- The baby is sleepy and reluctant to begin nursing or stay awake very long.
- You are nursing during the night.

You and your baby lie on your sides, tummy to tummy, as with the cuddle hold. Place your fingers beneath the breast and lift upward, then pull the baby in close after he roots with a wide open mouth.

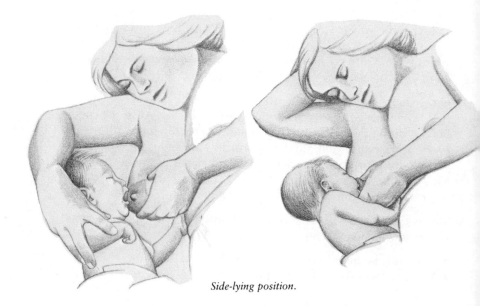

*Side-lying position.*

*Football hold.* The football hold is a terrific position when—

- You have had a cesarean birth and want to avoid placing the baby against your abdomen.
- You need more visibility in getting the baby to latch on.
- Your breasts are large.
- You are nursing a small baby, especially if he is premature.
- Your baby tends to slide down the areola onto the nipple.
- You are nursing twins.

The football hold offers you better control of the baby's head and greater visibility than other positions. One disadvantage is that you may have some trouble keeping the baby's hands and arms out of the way.

When you are getting started, a pillow at your side will help to support your elbow and the baby's bottom. Sit the baby up at your side at about the level of your waist, so he is facing you. Support his upper back with your arm, your hand holding his head at the level of your breast. With your other hand supporting the breast (fingers beneath and thumb above), stimulate the baby to root, and then pull him in close to latch on.

When you master one of these positions you should notice that very little or none of the areola is visible during nursing. This varies, of course, depending upon the size of the areola. Although you may feel some discomfort as the nipple stretches into the baby's mouth when he takes his first few sucks, nursing should be relatively comfortable thereafter. If it is not, take the baby off the breast and reposition him.

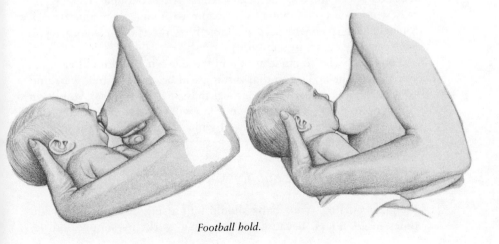

*Football hold.*

**Ending the feeding.** If the baby does not come off the breast by himself, and you want to switch breasts or rest awhile, you can take him off by first breaking the suction. Even if he is not actively sucking, his hold on the nipple is tremendously strong. To release the suction, pull down on his chin or insert your finger into the corner of his mouth, pushing your finger between his gums until you hear or feel the release.

After taking the baby off the breast, leave your bra flaps down so that the air can dry your nipples. Air drying helps to maintain healthy nipples.

**After a cesarean birth.** Whether or not your cesarean is planned, your milk will come in just as if you had delivered vaginally, and you can breastfeed your baby. Because you will be recovering from surgery, you will face some discomfort and possibly some difficulty maneuvering the baby to your breast. If you are expecting a cesarean, you may want to ask to share a hospital room with another woman who has had one. Some hospitals make such arrangements routinely.

If you are awake for your delivery, let the staff and the baby's physician know you wish to nurse as soon as possible. As long as the baby is not having any difficulties, there is no reason to delay nursing. If you can't sit up, you can nurse in the side-lying position with some help from your partner or the nurse.

If you are not fully conscious during the delivery, or if the baby is kept in the nursery by the doctor's orders, you can still begin nursing after your initial separation. Medication for pain is important for your comfort during the first few days; it will not hurt the baby. If you take the medication right after you nurse, moreover, a minimal amount will be in your milk at the next feeding. After a couple of days you may want to keep the baby in the room with you. Remember to ask for help whenever you need it. Sometimes the staff may forget you gave birth by cesarean section.

You may prefer to nurse at first in the side-lying position. Leave the side rails of the bed up so that turning will be easier. A pillow behind your back and one between your legs may be helpful. When you begin sitting up to nurse, a pillow on your lap will make you more comfortable. The football hold works well while sitting if you want to keep the baby off your abdomen.

## Insuring Your Milk Supply

**Frequent nursing.** Your baby should be nursing often, at least eight times in 24 hours. Because breastfeeding works by supply and demand, the more you nurse, the sooner your milk will come in, and the more milk you will have. After the first few days, most babies will want to nurse about every one to three hours. Breasts do not need to rest for any period of time to build up milk; it is constantly produced. The "good" baby who nurses every four hours (or less often) or who is sleeping through the night within the first few weeks is often the baby who fails to gain weight.

During the first few days after birth, many babies are sleepy. If your newborn has not nursed after three hours, unwrap her from her blankets, rub her back, and talk to her. She will probably then become interested in nursing.

In the hospital, keeping the baby with you in your room insures frequent nursing. If rooming-in is prohibited, ask the nurses to bring you the baby at least every three hours (more often if she fusses) and whenever she wakens during the night. In some hospitals, mothers go to the nursery to get their babies.

**Both breasts.** Encourage the baby to take both breasts at each feeding. When you hear her swallowing you will know that she is actively taking milk. When she has lost interest in the first breast or slowed her swallowing, (usually after about ten to twenty minutes), take her off and burp her: hold her against you with her head over your shoulder and gently rub her back, or sit her upright, bent slightly forward with your hand supporting her lower jaw, and firmly pat her lower back. After burping, she will probably regain interest in nursing and eagerly take the second breast. If she nurses only a short time or less vigorously at the second breast, start her on that side at the next feeding. This will encourage an even stimulation of both breasts.

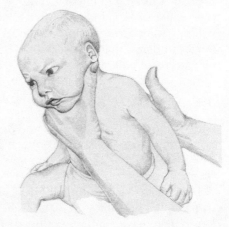

*You can burp the baby by sitting her up, one hand under her jaw. Firmly pat her back with the other hand.*

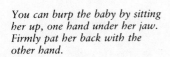

**Encouraging let-down.** An adequate milk supply depends on regular stimulation of the breasts. A baby gets most of the milk as the milk "lets down." You can encourage the let-down, and the production of more milk for the baby, by allowing her plenty of time to complete each feeding. Although some babies nurse for shorter or longer periods, most need ten to twenty minutes at each breast. Many mothers report that their milk lets down not just once but several times during a feeding. Limited feeding time, therefore, may not allow enough time to satisfy the baby and meet her growth demands.

Signs of milk let-down vary from woman to woman during the first week of nursing. Some new mothers experience mild uterine cramping and increased vaginal flow when the milk releases. Many, but not all, find their milk leaks, drips, or sprays during let-down. Very few women feel tingling in the breasts when the milk lets down, though most cannot recognize this sensation until after the first few weeks of nursing. In the meantime, probably the most reliable indicator of milk let-down is the sound of the baby swallowing.

While your baby is nursing, you can learn about your milk let-down. Typically, babies swallow in surges over a period of twenty minutes or so, or they swallow almost continuously for a lesser time. You can stimulate the milk to let down by gently massaging the breast as the baby nurses or by switching her from breast to breast several times during the feeding.

**Avoiding supplements.** Another way to insure your milk supply is to avoid supplemental feedings. Some babies become very confused when a bottle nipple is introduced during the first week (see Just the Breast). Glucose (sugar) water offers few calories and may discourage the baby's interest in nursing. (Also, a recent study has associated glucose water with jaundice.) After taking formula, a baby frequently will not want to nurse for four hours or longer, since formula takes longer to digest than breast milk. The decrease in breast stimulation may decrease milk production.

## The First Week of Nursing

Although most babies are alert and eager to nurse during the first two hours after birth, during the next few days they sleep most of the time. The average baby, after the first few days, begins to wake up on his own and wants to nurse about every one to three hours.

During nursing it is normal for a baby to suck a few times and then to pause. Some babies are "all-business" nursers; they seldom pause before they have emptied the breast or filled their stomachs. At the other extreme is the "dawdler," who pauses often; he may take from 40 to 60 minutes to complete a feeding.

While the baby is nursing you will hear him swallowing. Some babies gulp noisily (and may be swallowing lots of air); others are more quiet.

Clicking noises usually mean that the baby is not sucking adequately and therefore may not be receiving enough milk. The baby should have a strong enough hold on the breast so that it does not easily slip from his mouth. His cheeks should remain smooth with each suck; dimples on the cheek while nursing are a sign of inadequate suction and faulty sucking (see the Survival Guide for the First Week if your baby is having this problem).

During the first day babies sometimes spit up mucus they have swallowed during delivery. Occasionally a baby will gag on this mucus. After 24 hours, this is usually no longer a problem.

Babies often spit up colostrum or milk. The amounts are usually smaller than they seem, though parents may wonder if the baby is keeping anything down.

Babies also get hiccoughs, often after a feeding. If the baby starts hiccoughing after nursing at the first breast, it may be difficult to interest him in the other. You don't need to give him water or anything else. The hiccoughs are painless for him; just wait till they go away.

The baby's first stools, called meconium, are black and sticky, but his stools will become yellow soon after the milk is in, usually by the fifth or sixth day. The yellow stools are soft, loose or watery, and sometimes seedy. Babies normally strain and grunt when passing their stools—this does not mean they are constipated. Yellow stools passed daily usually indicate the baby is getting enough to eat.

Wet diapers are usually infrequent the first few days, but they will increase in number as the baby begins to get milk, usually by the fifth day. Eight or more diapers a day wet with pale urine are usually a sign of good milk intake. (This rule may not hold if the baby is receiving water.)

All newborns lose weight after birth. Your baby will probably lose about 5 to 10 percent of his birth weight.

**Caring for your breasts.** Your daily bath or shower is sufficient for cleaning your breasts. Avoid getting soap or shampoo on the nipple and areola; it tends to counteract the naturally occurring oils that cleanse this area. Antiseptic applications to the nipples are also unnecessary, but do take care to wash your hands before nursing.

You will probably want to wear a nursing bra for convenience and comfort, especially after your milk comes in. Again, bras with cotton rather than synthetic cups allow for better air circulation to the nipples.

If the baby does not come off the breast by herself when the nursing session is over, take care to release the suction with your finger. Leave your breasts exposed to the air for five or ten minutes before covering up. Air drying is soothing to the nipples.

Although for years mothers have used breast creams on their nipples, these do not prevent or reduce nipple soreness. In fact, a number of nursing women have developed sore nipples as a result of unsuspected allergies to preparations containing lanolin, vitamin E, or cocoa butter. Recently it was discovered that lanolin preparations were contaminated with residues of the pesticides with which sheep are sprayed. Any preparation that comes with instructions to wash it off before nursing is best avoided, as frequent washing is overly drying to the nipples. If you use a cream or oil, apply it sparingly around the nipple only.

Nursing pads are usually necessary during this time to prevent wet or spotted clothing. You can buy bra pads in two varieties: reusable, washable types, and disposable types. (Remember: if using a disposable pad, stay away from those with plastic liners because they keep the nipple wet and may aggravate soreness.)

If you are using plastic breast shells to improve the shape of your nipples, you may find during the first few weeks that they cause your milk to leak excessively and keep your nipples damp. You might try placing the shells in your bra just 20 to 30 minutes before the feeding (milk collected this way must be discarded). Don't routinely use breast shells in place of nursing pads; this would probably cause more leakage. Breast shells should be washed after each nursing in hot soapy water and rinsed thoroughly.

**When your milk comes in.** Milk production generally begins on the second or third day postpartum, but occasionally not until the fourth or fifth day. Mother's milk is whiter than colostrum but more watery looking than cow's milk; it often resembles skim milk.

Most women notice that their breasts become larger, fuller, and more tender as the milk comes in. This change, known as engorgement, is caused by increased blood flow to the breasts as well as beginning milk production. Fullness may be more apparent if your breasts are normally small or medium-sized. They may feel lumpy, and the lumpiness may extend all the way to your armpits, as milk glands are also located there.

Putting your baby to breast you may feel any of these normal sensations: warmth, relaxation, sleepinesss, thirst, and even hunger.

During this time it is normal for milk to leak from the breasts. When the baby nurses at one breast, milk may drip from the other. This leaking may continue for several weeks, or it may never happen at all.

Engorgement normally lasts 24 to 48 hours. During this time a nursing bra will provide comfort and support. Frequent nursing, at least every two to three hours, is the best treatment. Engorgement may be further relieved by gently massaging the breast while the baby is nursing. This will encourage more milk to let down. It is important to pay careful attention to the way the baby latches on while the breast is engorged. When latch-on is incorrect because the baby isn't positioned well or the areola is overly full, soreness often follows. If the areola is hard, you can express some milk, by hand or with a pump, until it has softened enough to permit the baby to latch on properly.

(For further advice on managing engorgement, see the Survival Guide for the First Week.)

**From hospital to home.** At the time of discharge it is customary in many hospitals to give new mothers an array of sample products that manufacturers would like them to try. It may appear that the staff endorses these products; it doesn't necessarily. One of these gifts is usually a package of formula, sometimes called a "breastfeeding kit." The "kit" contains formula, bottle nipples, and a pamplet on breastfeeding. These pamphlets sometimes contain misleading information about nursing. Since you have chosen to breastfeed, it is best to leave the kit behind. You won't be needing it.

What are well worth taking home, however, are the names and numbers of people who have a good reputation for helping nursing mothers and infants. Ask the nurse who was encouraging or helpful with your early breastfeeding for this information. She may know of volunteers in La Leche League or the Nursing Mothers Counsel, or lactation professionals in your community.

*At home.* As any experienced nursing mother can tell you, the first few days at home with a baby are exhausting and, at times, emotional. These days are best spent caring only for yourself and the baby. Besides recovering from the birth, you are doing the important work of getting to know your baby and learning to breastfeed. Rest and a quiet, pleasant environment are important in preventing anxiety, or "baby blues." Try to eat well, but don't worry if your appetite has lessened; this can be normal during the first couple of weeks after delivery. Ideally, you should spend the first several days nursing and resting with the baby, while a supportive partner or helper (or both) manages your home, meals, any other children, and callers.

It is not uncommon for things to suddenly "fall apart" shortly after a new mother comes home from the hospital. Suddenly responsible for a new baby, you may feel shaky at times and your confidence may vanish. The dramatic hormonal shift that begins immediately after birth may also affect your emotional state for a short time. You may find yourself exhausted and upset—especially if you've been taking responsibility for more than the baby and yourself.

The postpartum period is a time of physical and emotional adjustment. As with most changes in life, it is usually accompanied by some turmoil. It will take several weeks, and most of your time and energy, to get to know your baby and learn how to care for him. So don't do more than you must, and accept offers for help. Adjusting to motherhood is always easier when you are supported and cared for by others.

# SURVIVAL GUIDE
## for the First Week

### Concerns About Yourself

Engorged Breasts

Sore Nipples

Breast Pain

Leaking Milk

Let-down Difficulty

Milk Appearance

Difficult Latch-on: Flat, Dimpled, or Inverted Nipples

Fatigue and Depression

### Concerns About the Baby

Sleepy Baby

Bowel Movements

Jaundice

Difficult Latch-on: Refusal to Nurse

Sucking Problems

Fussiness and Excessive Night Waking

Underfeeding and Weight Loss

# Concerns About Yourself

## *Engorged Breasts*

At two or three days postpartum the breasts usually become engorged, or temporarily swollen and uncomfortable. This is caused by the increased flow of blood to the breasts and the start of milk production. For some women the breasts become only slightly full, but for others they feel very swollen, tender, throbbing, and lumpy. Sometimes the swelling extends all the way to the armpit. Engorgement may cause the nipple to flatten, making it difficult for the baby to latch on. The problem usually lessens within 24 to 48 hours, but the swelling and discomfort may worsen if nursing is too brief or infrequent.

Although many health care providers recommend applying direct heat (warm washcloths, heating pads, hot water bottles, or hot showers) to engorged breasts, this may actually aggravate engorgement.

**Treatment measures for engorged breasts**

1. Wear a supportive nursing bra, even during the night. Be sure your bra is not too tight.

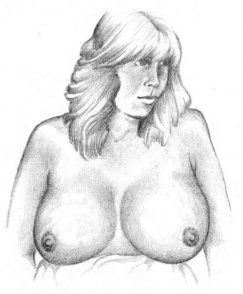

*The breasts may grow astonishingly big and hard as milk production begins.*

2. Nurse frequently, every one to three hours, and use both breasts at each feeding. This may mean waking the baby (see Sleepy Baby.).

3. Avoid having the baby latch on when the areola is very firm. To reduce the possibility of damage to your nipples, manually express or pump milk until the areola softens. It may be easier to manually express milk in the shower; the warm water by itself may cause enough leakage to soften the areola. Wearing plastic breast shells for half an hour before nursing also helps to soften the areola.

4. Encourage the baby to nurse 10 to 20 minutes or longer at each breast.

5. Gently massage the breast at which the baby is nursing. This will encourage the milk to flow and will help relieve some of the tightness and discomfort you feel.

6. To soothe the pain and help relieve swelling, apply cold packs to the breast for a short period *after* nursing. Crushed ice in a plastic bag works well.

7. If you need to, take acetaminophen tablets (such as Tylenol) or a mild pain reliever prescribed by your doctor.

8. Avoid pumping milk except when you need to soften the areola or when the baby refuses the second breast. Excessive or habitual pumping can lead to overproduction of milk.

## Sore Nipples

There is no doubt about it: sore nipples can make a trial of what ought to be a joyous experience. For a few days after giving birth, you may feel slight tenderness during the first minute of nursing, when the baby latches on and the nipple stretches into her mouth. Such tenderness is normal at this time. (See the General Comfort Measures for Sore Nipples).

If your nipples become really sore, however, they are probably damaged or irritated and require treatment beyond simple comfort measures. It is important for you to identify the cause of the problem so that you can help your nipples heal. At any time that you are unable to tolerate the pain, and the position changes recommended in the following pages do not help, consult a lactation professional. If none is available, you may want to stop nursing; manually express or pump your milk for 24 to 72 hours, or until the nipples heal (see Chapter 5 on manually expressing and pumping milk).

*Identifying the problem.* There are two basic types of sore nipples: the traumatized nipple and the irritated nipple. The traumatized nipple may be blistered, scabbed, or cracked. The irritated nipple is very pink and often burns. Occasionally a mother may have both types of soreness at the same time.

| If you have— | See— |
|---|---|
| Tenderness, blisters, or scabs on the end of the nipple | Injured Tips |
| Tenderness or cracks at the base of the nipple | Chewed Nipples, Thrush Nipples, Irritated Nipples |
| Soreness only below the nipple | Soreness on the Underside of the Nipples |
| Burning, red nipples | Thrush Nipples, Irritated Nipples |
| Burning, itching, flaking, oozing, or crusting areola and nipple | Eczema |

**Injured tips.** These nipples are tender, bruised, scabbed, or blistered *on the tip*. The damage results when the nipple enters the baby's mouth at a upward angle and rubs against the roof of his mouth. This can happen if you sit leaning back to nurse (as in a hospital bed), if your latch-on technique is incorrect (see Chapter 2), or if the nipple points upward naturally.

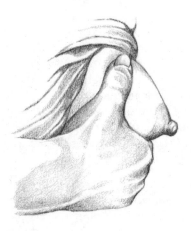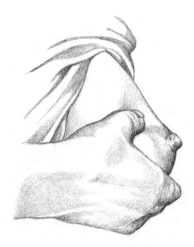

*Aim the nipple down, not up, as the baby latches on.*

**Treatment measures for injured tips**

1. If your breast is so full that the areola cannot be easily compressed, manually express or pump enough milk to soften the areola. This will make it easier for the baby to latch on and may help stimulate the milk to let down. The baby should then get down to business sooner, and finish sooner as well.
2. Sit up straight so that the nipple points straight out or downward.
3. Position the baby and the breast carefully. The football or the cross-cuddle hold is highly recommended (see Chapter 2). Be sure to lift the breast upward so the nipple points downward. Avoid pressing the top of the breast with your thumb or index finger.
4. Review the General Comfort Measures for Sore Nipples.

**Chewed nipples.** These are tender or cracked *at or near the base,* where the nipple connects to the areola. "Nipple chewing" usually results because a baby is improperly positioned for nursing; her gums close on the nipple instead of the areola. This can also occur when a baby refuses to open her mouth wide enough or when her gums slide off the areola onto the nipple, commonly when the breast is engorged or not supported. Cracking may also occur with irritated nipples and thrush nipples; (see the sections on both).

Some babies who are "tongue-tied" can also make the base of the nipples sore as they nurse (see the section on "tongue-tied" babies under Difficult Latch-on, later in this Survival Guide).

**Treatment measures for chewed nipples**

1. If your breast is so full that the areola cannot be easily compressed, manually express or pump enough milk to soften the areola. This will allow the baby to get more of the areola into her mouth and will help to stimulate let-down.
2. Position the baby and the breast carefully (see Chapter 2). The football or the cross-cuddle hold is highly recommended. Keep your fingers off the areola; just wait for the baby to open her mouth wide, then pull her in very close. The baby should be pulled in so close that her nose is momentarily buried in the breast.
3. Use the football or the cross-cuddle hold to control the position of the baby's head through the entire feeding. This will allow you to prevent her gums from sliding down onto the nipple after she has latched on.
4. If your baby is reluctant to open her mouth wide, don't let her chew her way onto the breast. Patiently wait until she opens her mouth. Letting the baby suck on your finger for a few seconds may encourage her to open more enthusiastically.
5. Do not hesitate to take the baby off the breast as soon as you realize that she is not in the right position. You may need to help her latch on several times before you succeed at getting her far enough onto the breast. Ask your partner, helper, or lactation professional to observe your latch-on

technique. A helper can also guide your arm when the baby opens wide so that she is pulled in as close as possible.

6. Review the General Comfort Measures for Sore Nipples.

**Soreness on the underside of the nipples.** This is usually caused by the baby who is nursing with his bottom lip tucked in. Normally the lip should turn out. When the bottom lip is tucked in, it rubs against the underside of the nipple, causing a friction burn.

Pull the baby's lower lip out while he is nursing; this will usually relieve the pain immediately. You may need to do this several times during the nursing session.

Review the General Comfort Measures for Sore Nipples.

**Irritated nipples (nipple dermatitis).** Irritated nipples are reddened and sometimes slightly swollen, and *generally they burn.* Some mothers may feel burning between as well as during feedings. In severe cases, the nipples may be cracked. Nipple dermatitis is most commonly caused by an allergic response to a nipple cream or oil.

Common offenders are vitamin E preparations—oils, creams, or capsules. Lanolin may also cause an allergic response, usually in a mother who is allergic to wool (from which lanolin comes) or very sensitive to it. Lanolin is found in pure hydrous or anhydrous form and in many commercial creams, such as Masse Cream, Mammol Ointment, Eucerin, and A & D Ointment. Mothers allergic to chocolate may develop an allergic reaction to preparations with cocoa butter, such as Balm Barr.

Simply discontinuing use of the cream or oil may bring some relief, but usually additional measures are necessary.

**Treatment measures for irritated nipples**

1. Call your doctor, who may prescribe an anti-inflammatory preparation. If the doctor is reluctant, you may want to see a dermatologist.

2. Place cool, wet compresses on the nipples after nursing.

3. Apply the medication to the irritated areas after every other nursing, making sure your nipples are completely dry first. The cream should be applied sparingly so that all of it is absorbed. If you see traces on your nipples when you are ready to nurse again, you are using too much. Dab. the area with a tissue to absorb the excess.

4. Use the medication for as long as advised by your doctor. Although the pain may be gone in a day or two, the dermatitis may take from two to three weeks to completely heal.

5. Should you find that the medication aggravates your soreness, stop using it immediately. This may indicate that yeast is present and should be treated. (See Thrush Nipples, below.)

6. Review the General Comfort Measures for Sore Nipples.

**Thrush nipples.** This problem occurs when a yeast *(monilia)* infection in the baby's mouth spreads to the mother's nipples. The nipples become reddened, swollen, tender, and sometimes cracked. Occasionally white curds can be seen on the nipples. Some mothers complain of itching and flaking; others complain of burning.

When a mother's nipples become sore after weeks or months of comfortable nursing, thrush is the usual cause. But a thrush infection may also occur in the first weeks after delivery, and when it does it may be overlooked as the cause of the nipple soreness. A newborn with thrush may have picked up a yeast infection in the birth canal during delivery; this often happens if the mother is diabetic. A thrush infection may also result if a mother or her baby is given antibiotics (after a cesarean, antibiotics are often given in intravenous fluids).

If you suspect a case of thrush, carefully inspect the baby's mouth. You may see white patches on the tongue, cheeks, insides of the lips, or gums. Sometimes a baby will have no symptoms in the mouth but will have a diaper rash caused by yeast. This rash often resembles a mild burn; it may peel and does not respond to ordinary measures. Sometimes the rash looks like just a patch of red dots.

### Treatment measures for thrush nipples

1. Both the mother and the baby must be treated in order to prevent reinfection. The treatment usually recommended is 1 milliliter of nystatin suspension (Mycostatin) by dropper into the baby's mouth after every other nursing, or four times daily, for 14 days. Half the dose should be dropped into each side of the mouth. For the nipples, nystatin ointment is recommended;

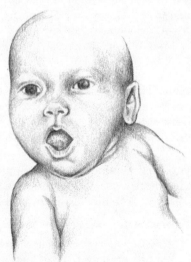

*Thrush often appears as white, cheesy patches on the baby's tongue or on the insides of the cheeks.*

the baby's medicine can also be used, but it may be less effective. The medication should be applied after each nursing. In either form, nystatin must be prescribed by a physician. Store it in the refrigerator, and, even though the symptoms may be gone after a few days, continue the treatment for the full 14 days.

Another treatment that is sometimes recommended is swabbing the baby's mouth and the mother's nipples with a 1 percent solution of gentian violet, which can be purchased at most drugstores without a prescription. Thoroughly swab the affected areas in the baby's mouth, and your nipples and areola, with a cotton-tipped applicator once or twice a day for three days. The solution will stain the baby's mouth and your breasts purple; take care in applying so that nothing else turns purple.

2. If you are using nystatin, it is best to wait for 15 minutes after nursing before giving it to the baby so it isn't washed out of her system with the milk. Some counselors also recommend rinsing your nipples after each nursing the first few days with water or a mild solution of vinegar (one tablespoon vinegar to one cup water) before applying the cream or drops.

3. In addition to medication, brief exposure to the sun two or three times daily may hasten the healing of the nipples.

4. Changing the nursing pads at each feeding is a must to prevent reinfection.

5. Pacifiers, rubber nipples, and plastic breast shells must be boiled for 20 minutes every day during treatment. If you are using nystatin, these nipples should be replaced at the end of the first week.

6. If you are using a pump, it is important to wash all pump parts thoroughly after each use. In addition, the parts that come in contact with the breast or the milk should be boiled for 20 minutes daily.

7. If nystatin suspension has not cleared thrush from your baby's mouth after five to six days of treament, try using gentian violet (as described in item 1) in addition to the nystatin.

8. If your nipples are not significantly better after several days of the treatment just described, see a dermatologist for additional treatment.

**Eczema.** This condition can appear on the nipple and areola, making the area burn, itch, flake, ooze, or crust. Women with a history or current outbreak of eczema elsewhere on the body are most often affected. Treatment from a dermatologist should be sought.

Try to keep in mind that your nipples won't be sore forever. The following measures, in addition to the specific treatments listed for each category of sore nipples, will speed healing and provide comfort.

**General comfort measures for sore nipples**

1. Take acetaminophen tablets (such as Tylenol) or a pain reliever prescribed by your doctor, a half-hour before nursing.

2. Express a small amount of milk just before the baby latches on.

3. Apply ice to the nipple just before the baby latches on.

4. Begin nursing on the least sore side (if there is one).

5. Avoid nipple shields for nursing. These often make the soreness worse, and they may decrease your milk supply.

6. Massage your breasts while nursing to encourage the milk to flow and to speed emptying.

7. Restrict nursing time to about ten minutes per side if you are sore during the entire feeding. This will probably mean nursing more often (every hour or two).

8. Release the baby's suction hold carefully before removing the baby from the breast.

9. Air-dry the nipples after each feeding. Leave the nipples exposed to the air as much as possible between nursings. A cotton T-shirt worn without a bra, or with your bra flaps down, will provide good air circulation to the nipples.

10. Don't apply nipple creams or tea bags to your nipples. These do not reduce nipple pain or necessarily promote healing.

11. Change nursing pads after each nursing and when they become wet. Make sure there are no plastic liners hidden in the pads; cut them open and check if you are not absolutely sure.

12. Wear cotton bras. Other fabrics do not allow adequate air circulation.

13. Wash plastic breast shells daily, if you use them at all. Shells may prevent the nipples from rubbing against your bra, but they may also encourage dripping, keep the nipples moist, and delay healing.

14. Avoid excessive washing of your nipples. Rinse them in your daily bath or shower, but avoid getting soap on them. Do take care to wash your hands before handling your breasts.

15. Leave scabs and blisters alone.

16. Do not delay nursings. Shorter, more frequent nursings (every hour to three hours) are easier on the nipples.

17. If you are using a breast pump during a period of soreness, pump your milk often—at least eight times a day—to keep your supply maintained. Be sure to use the correct size shield for your nipple, and carefully center it before starting to pump (see Chapter 5).

## Breast Pain

You may feel pain in your breasts if you become engorged, which usually happens two to four days after delivery (see Engorged Breasts).

Occasionally mothers complain of breast pain while nursing. If you feel a burning pain and your nipples are pinker than normal, refer to Thrush Nipples and Irritated Nipples. If you feel a mild aching at the start of nursing, it is probably related to the beginning of let-down.

A deep pain, sometimes described as "shooting," that occurs soon after nursing is believed to be related to the sudden refilling of the breast. This discomfort is usually temporary and disappears after the first weeks of nursing.

## Leaking Milk

During the early weeks of nursing, milk may drip, leak or spray from the breasts. This is a normal sign of let-down. While the baby nurses at one breast, milk often drips or sprays from the other. Let-down, and leaking, may occur frequently and unexpectedly between nursings as well. Milk may leak during sleep. It may be stimulated by the baby's sounds, by thoughts about nursing, or by any routines associated with feeding time. A shower may stimulate let-down. Dripping, leaking, and spraying usually lessen considerably after a few weeks of nursing.

Some mothers' breasts do not leak. Mothers who have nursed previously may notice that their breasts leak less with subsequent children. Both of these situations are usually normal.

**Coping measures for leaking milk**

1. Open both bra flaps while nursing and let the milk drip into a small towel or diaper.
2. Change nursing pads as soon as they become wet. Avoid those with plastic liners.
3. Avoid routine use of plastic breast shells if you do not need them to improve the shape of your nipples. They may keep your clothes dry, but they can cause excessive leaking and keep your nipples moist. Milk collected in the shells between nursings is unsafe for feeding. Only if the shells are boiled just prior to nursing and put in place during nursing can the milk be stored for later feedings.
4. Pumping your breasts will not control leaking. In fact, it will stimulate greater milk production and possibly make your breasts fuller and more prone to leaking.
5. Place extra pads in your bra if your breasts leak during the night. You may want to spread a bath towel over the bed sheet to eliminate middle-of-the-night linen changes and to protect your mattress.
6. Do not try to stop leaking with the pressure of your fingers or forearm during the first weeks, since this may inhibit milk let-down and may possibly lead to plugged milk ducts.

## Let-down Difficulty

During the early weeks of breastfeeding, the let-down response is developing. Sometimes mothers are told that they must be happy, relaxed, and carefree for the let-down of milk to occur. If this were the case, few women would ever succeed at nursing. Although many mothers worry that their milk won't be available as needed, let-down failure is extremely rare among women who nurse regularly and often.

For the establishment and maximal functioning of the let-down reflex, nurse the baby every two to three hours around the clock during the first week. Make sure that she is positioned correctly and is compressing the sinuses beneath the areola, and that her feeding time is not limited. Ideally, the baby should be allowed—encouraged, if necessary—to nurse at least 10 to 20 minutes at each breast.

It is also important that you are as comfortable as possible. The milk may not release completely if you are experiencing much pain— whether from sore nipples or from the trauma of delivery.

The signs of milk release during the first week will vary for each woman. They *may* include—

- mild uterine cramping during nursing;
- increased vaginal flow during nursing;
- dripping, leaking, or spraying of milk, especially during nursing;
- occasional sensations in the breast during nursing (usually not felt during the first week); and
- softening of the breasts after nursing (this may not be noticeable during the period of initial engorgement, two to four days postpartum).

The most reliable indicator of milk let-down is the sound of the baby swallowing. As the milk releases the baby will swallow after every couple of sucks. A typical rhythm is suck-suck-suck-swallow-suck-suck-swallow. The swallowing pattern may occur steadily over several minutes or may come in surges of two or three minutes at a time.

The signs of a sluggish let-down usually include *all* of the following:

- no cramping;
- no leaking of milk;
- no sign of the breasts softening after nursing; and
- no swallowing, or swallowing during only the first minute or two of nursing (the baby may then swallow only occasionally or pull away from the breast crying).

Not infrequently when a mother believes she is experiencing a let-down difficulty, the problem is actually with the baby's latch-on or sucking.

### Treatment measures for let-down difficulty

1. Nurse regularly, frequently, and for as long as the baby wants.
2. Make yourself as comfortable as possible before nursing. Take a pain reliever at least a half-hour before nursing if you need it. Nurse in a relaxing place.

3. Before nursing, apply moist heat to your breasts and spend several minutes gently massaging them.

4. Try manually expressing or pumping a small amount of milk to encourage the flow to begin.

5. Carefully position the baby at your breast. Take care that the baby is pulled in very close (see Chapter 2). The football hold may help the baby nurse more efficiently.

6. Make sure the baby is latching on and sucking correctly. She should have a strong, steady suction while nursing, and you should not hear frequent clicking noises or see dimples in her cheeks. (See Difficult Latch-on: Refusal to Nurse, and Sucking Problems.)

7. Massage your breasts during the entire feeding, and practice slow, deep breathing.

8. Switch breasts if you do not hear swallowing within five minutes. Continue switching breasts every five minutes if swallowing is infrequent.

9. Ask for outside help if you still are not hearing swallowing after a few feedings. Seeing a lactation professional may be helpful. Your physician may prescribe oxytocin (Syntocinon) nasal spray for you. The 5-milliliter size costs around thirty dollars. Spray the oxytocin once or twice in one nostril three to four minutes before every nursing. After a day or two, the let-down will probably be working on its own. Rarely is a second bottle necessary.

## Milk Appearance

Whereas colostrum is usually clear, yellow, or orange, mature breast milk is white, sometimes with a bluish tint. If it resembles skim milk from the dairy, this does not mean your milk is "weak"; breast milk normally looks thin. Occasionally a mother discovers that her milk is green, blue, or pink. Such coloring is due to her intake of vegetables, fruits, food dyes, or dietary supplements, and is not harmful to the baby.

Blood in the milk can usually be traced to a bleeding nipple. Occasionally bleeding from the breast occurs during pregnancy or when breastfeeding begins. Frequently, a benign papilloma is the cause, and the bleeding generally stops within several days. Blood in the milk will not hurt the baby, though substantial amounts may make him vomit. If you are advised against nursing, ask if you can pump awhile to see if it clears up on its own.

## Difficult Latch-on: Flat, Dimpled, or Inverted Nipples

Both mother and baby get frustrated when latching on to the breasts is difficult because of flat, dimpled, or inverted nipples. Typically, the problem is intensified if the breasts become engorged or overly full.

When they do, even nipples that seemed normal may suddenly flatten or dimple. Frequently, one nipple proves to be more troublesome than the other. Persistence and patience help most mothers through this problem.

Mothers with problem nipples are often more prone to soreness. This is because latch-on becomes their number-one priority; they give little attention to correct positioning.

### Treatment measures for flat, dimpled, or inverted nipples

1. Put the baby to the breast within the first two hours after birth. The timing of the first nursing may be critical when the nipples are flat, dimpled, or inverted. A great number of babies are able to latch on easily to problem nipples during this initial period, and they continue to do well.

2. Avoid giving the baby an artificial nipple of any kind. Whether or not your baby succeeded at latching on at first try, this is very important. An artificial nipple often makes his subsequent attempts more difficult.

3. Stimulate the nipples to help them stand out, by gently stroking or rolling them between your thumb and forefinger. Or, apply ice to the nipple just before the baby attempts to latch on.

4. To help the baby latch on, make a flat nipple stand out by pinching it between your thumb and forefinger. This won't work with a dimpled or inverted nipple, which will invert further when pinched. Instead, place your thumb about one and a half to two inches behind the nipple, with your fingers beneath, and pull back toward your chest. The football hold will allow you the most visibility and control.

5. Wear breast shells in your bra at least a half-hour before nursing if your breasts are engorged—this is often essential for dimpled or inverted nipples. Many hospital maternity units have breast shells. If yours doesn't, send your partner or friend to any maternity shop for a pair. (See Planning for the First Days, Chapter 1.)

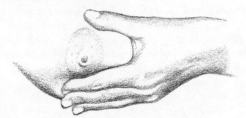

*To help the baby latch on to an inverted nipple, place your thumb above the areola and your fingers below, and push your breast against your chest wall.*

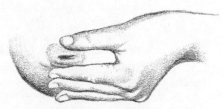

*Don't squeeze your thumb and forefinger together, or the nipple may invert further.*

6. Pump your breasts just before nursing to pull the nipples out enough for the baby to latch on. Any pump can be used for this.

7. Express a few drops of colostrum or milk onto your nipple or onto the baby's lips if he is reluctant to latch on. Glucose water dripped over the nipple may also entice the baby, although it sometimes makes the nipple too slippery. (*Never* use honey or corn syrup on your nipple, as they have been associated with infant botulism.)

8. Stop nursing if the baby is frantic, and calm him for awhile. Dripping glucose water on his lips also helps to calm him and gain his interest in latching on.

9. If a nurse or another helper is working with you, use the side-lying position to allow your helper maximum visibility and control. If your nipples are dimpled or inverted, ask the helper to pull back on the breast behind the nipple; pinching will usually result in further inversion. Sometimes these sessions become intense and upsetting, so let your helper know when you or your baby needs a break. If you are in the hospital, let a variety of nurses work with you; you can usually find one or two who are exceptionally skilled and sensitive.

10. Refuse any offers from nurses of rubber nipple shields or bottle nipples to place over your own nipple for nursing. Your baby will latch on and suck, but the shield does not allow for adequate stimulation of your nipple, or for the necessary compression of the sinuses beneath the areola. The shield can thus inhibit the let-down of milk and adequate emptying of the breast, possibly leading to a poor milk supply and insufficient milk intake for the baby. In addition, most babies who begin nursing with a rubber nipple shield will refuse to ever nurse without it.

If you do choose to try this method to make your nipples stand out, wait until at least 24 hours after birth to give the baby a chance to nurse on his own. Take off the shield after one to two minutes of sucking, and attempt latch-on without it. Pumping just prior to nursing accomplishes the same thing.

11. Begin bottle feedings after 24 to 48 hours if your baby still has not latched on. Use a Nuk or similarly shaped nipple; these are widely available in drugstores. An electric pump is usually the best choice for collecting milk and improving the nipple shape. Continue putting the baby to breast.

12. Occasionally a mother and her baby are discharged from the hospital before nursing has occurred. If this happens to you, locate an electric pump (see Appendix A) and use it at least eight times a day (see Chapter 3 for guidelines on pumping). Keep trying to nurse; once at home, short practice sessions at least three to four times per day, on a soft breast when the baby is not frantic, eventually pay off. In this situation you may need a great deal of support and encouragement. Finding this support will make all the difference. Seeing a lacation professional may be very helpful. It is very common for the baby to suddenly latch on one day, rewarding your persistence.

## Fatigue and Depression

During this first week, make your life as simple as possible. Your partner or helper is essential, of course, to your recovery and adjustment. He or she can be most helpful in assuring your rest by taking over family and household duties and limiting phone calls and visitors.

Rest is necessary to your ability to cope during the postpartum period. Make a commitment to take at least one nap a day, to make up for sleep lost in labor and afterward, due to frequent feeding demands. You may find that you are able to sleep better during naps and at night if you tuck the baby in with you. Babies often sleep better this way too. An answering machine can be very helpful in preventing disruptions while you nap. It's also handy when you are busy with nursing and baby care.

Eat a good breakfast—perhaps your partner can prepare it for you. If you lack an appetite at mealtimes, frequent snacking throughout the day on high-protein foods will assist your own physical recovery and help maintain your energy level.

If you have had tearing or an episiotomy, or you have hemorrhoids, take several baths each day. Warm water is soothing and relaxing, and it will speed healing of your perineum.

Don't expect yourself to adjust to new parenthood on your own. Reach out for help or reassurance whenever you need it. Friends or relatives might welcome the opportunity to come and help out for a while, and you should feel free to call the hospital staff, a public health nurse, your childbirth instructor, or a breastfeeding counselor whenever you need assistance, reassurance, or support.

If you feel tired and overwhelmed, try not to keep it to yourself. Let your partner know—a good cry on someone's shoulder may leave you feeling much better. Avoid making your partner the target of your fears and anger; instead of criticizing, let him know exactly what you need. One mother put it very well: "I just need him to give me hugs and let me know I'm doing OK." Your partner, after all, may be feeling as much stress as you are.

Feeling depressed over a birth experience is not uncommon. You may be able to resolve some of your feelings by talking to your childbirth instructor or birth attendant. In a week or two, you might try to locate a postpartum or cesarean support group.

If you are alone with your baby during this first week, make a special effort to continue limiting your activities. Perhaps you can have a friend come by to fix you lunch. Let the dishes soak all day, and pick up the house for only ten minutes at a time, if you must. Unplug the phone and place a sign on your door when it's time for your nap. Perhaps you can afford to pay for light housekeeping once or twice a week for a short period.

# Concerns about the Baby

## *Sleepy Baby*

Most babies are sleepy during the first several days after birth. They may be so sleepy that they refuse to nurse or they fall asleep after just a few minutes of nursing. Sleepiness the first few days may be related in part to recovery following labor and delivery. Medications and anesthetics given to the mother during the birth process also lessen the baby's wakefulness and interest in nursing. When newborns are wrapped snugly, too, they usually sleep for long periods of time (that's why nurses bundle them tightly). Babies may act too sleepy to nurse when they feel full from water or formula supplements—or an air bubble. The newborn with jaundice may also be somewhat sleepy.

Although it may seem unkind, the sleepy baby should be wakened and fed at least every three hours. The sleepy baby needs a "mother-led" rather than a "demand" schedule until she begins waking on her own. This is necessary not only for her nutritional well-being but to insure milk production and supply. Frequent feedings will also help minimize jaundice.

**Treatment measures for the sleepy baby**

1. Attempt nursing only after waking the baby. This is best accomplished by unwrapping and undressing her down to the diaper. Dim any bright lights, and sit the baby up on your lap by holding her under her chin. While talking to the baby, gently rub or pat her back (you may even get a burp).
2. Stroke the baby's forehead with a cool (not cold) wash cloth to help waken the very persistent sleeper.
3. If the baby falls back asleep soon after latching on, use the side-lying position to encourage her to nurse for longer periods. You may need assistance from someone else to get the baby to latch on. The football hold may also be helpful in keeping the baby awake, though not as effective as side-lying nursing.
4. Burp the baby after nursing at one breast to encourage her to take the other. Sitting the baby up in your lap and bending her slightly forward usually works best. Change her diaper if needed.
5. Be persistent. If all else fails, which may happen, try again in a half-hour.
6. Avoid supplements, pacifiers, and rubber nipple shields. All of these increase the baby's reluctance to nurse.

7. While in the hospital, take advantage of the baby's normal sleeping waking cycles by keeping the baby with you as much as possible.

8. Alert your physician if your baby is very lethargic and cannot be roused by the preceding techniques after five to six hours.

## Bowel Movements

Your baby's first few stools are called meconium. Meconium is black, greenish-black, or dark brown, and is tarry or sticky. By the second or third day, after several good colostrum feedings, the baby will have passed most of the meconium; he may have a few greenish-brown or brownish-yellow transitional stools.

Once milk production is established and the baby is nursing well, stools take on their characteristic color of yellow or mustard. This usually occurs by the fifth or sixth day. If the baby does not nurse well during the first couple of days or if he becomes jaundiced, his stools may remain darker for another day or two. The yellow stool is a sign that the baby is getting a sufficient amount of milk.

During the early days most babies have at least one bowel movement daily; many have several. The stools of a breastfed baby are generally the consistency of yogurt. They are soft and may even be runny; they may appear curdled or seedy. This is not diarrhea. These stools have a sweet or cheesy odor.

Your baby may pass his stools easily, or he may fuss, grunt, and turn red in the face while having a bowel movement. This is not constipation. Constipation is not possible as long as your baby is totally breastfed.

## Jaundice

A yellowing of the skin and eyes, jaundice is caused by bilirubin, a yellow pigment that is present to some degree in all blood. The skin becomes yellowish when the amount of bilirubin is higher than normal.

Bilirubin comes from the red blood cells. These cells live only a short time; as they are destroyed bilirubin is made. Bilirubin is then processed through the liver and finally eliminated in the stool. During pregnancy, the mother's liver processes bilirubin for the baby. After birth, the baby's liver has to learn to do the job. This usually takes a few days. Until the baby's liver is able to process bilirubin, it may increase in the baby's blood. This normal rise is referred to as physiologic jaundice. This is the most common form of jaundice, and about

40 percent of all babies develop it. It is usually noticed on the second or third day of life, and it generally disappears by one week of age.

Mild to moderate jaundice of this type will not hurt a baby, although many parents worry about it. Nor is the condition more frequent or serious among breastfed babies, as commonly believed. However, the baby who nurses poorly or not at all during the first few days may become jaundiced from the lack of colostrum, which is important for the elimination of meconium. When meconium is retained in the bowel longer than usual, bilirubin cannot be eliminated as needed. The best way of treating this jaundice is by nursing often.

Some babies develop jaundice for other reasons. One type of jaundice, ABO incompatability, occurs when the mother's blood type is O and the baby's blood type is A, B, or AB. During pregnancy, maternal antibodies cross the placenta, break down red blood cells, and cause more bilirubin to be produced in the baby after birth. On the first or second day after delivery, the bilirubin level may rise rapidly. Other, less common blood incompatibilities also produce elevated bilirubin levels.

Babies with any bruises resulting from the birth process commonly develop jaundice. Also more prone to jaundice are babies who are sick right after birth or born premature, at low birth weights, or to diabetic mothers. Twins, too, are especially susceptible. Some drugs that are used during labor can also cause jaundice.

An unusual type of jaundice, known as breast-milk jaundice, occurs in approximately one in two hundred fifty nursing babies. Breast-milk jaundice does not generally appear until the fifth day after birth. It usually lasts four to six weeks but can continue for as long as eight to ten weeks. The exact cause of this jaundice is still unknown, but it has never been known to cause any problem for a baby. When a baby's skin stays yellow beyond the first week, breast-milk jaundice is diagnosed by discontinuing nursing for 12 to 24 hours. The bilirubin level usually drops dramatically, after which breastfeeding can be safely resumed. The bilirubin level usually rises gradually again. Interestingly, if the mother nurses a second baby, the chance of reoccurrence is about 75 percent.

If your baby looks jaundiced, the doctor may order tests to measure the level of bilirubin in the blood and determine whether treatment is necessary. If the baby was born at term and is otherwise healthy, many doctors will not order treatment unless the bilirubin level is over 14 or 15 milligrams. Frequent breastfeeding may be all that is necessary.

Some babies may be treated with phototherapy. The "bili-lights," along with frequent nursing, help to destroy excess bilirubin. The baby usually lies under these lights from two to four days, her eyes covered with a protective mask. Often, the bilirubin level will stay constant for 24 hours and drop by 48 hours. The treatment is discontinued as soon as the bilirubin level has dropped to a normal level. Usually a baby is hospitalized for phototherapy, but in some communities home phototherapy services are available.

Rarely, usually in cases of blood incompatability, the bilirubin climbs rapidly to high levels. On these occasions an exchange transfusion may be done to reduce the bilirubin. Over an hour or two, small amounts of the baby's blood are taken out and replaced with donated blood.

Some doctors ask the mother to stop breastfeeding temporarily whenever a baby becomes jaundiced. This is usually unnecessary, since breast milk is rarely the cause of jaundice; indeed, many physicians believe that breastfeeding is one of the most effective ways of eliminating it. Calling a halt to nursing is also unfortunate for the mother, who may wonder if her milk is really best for her baby.

Mothers are also commonly told that their nursing babies need water supplements to help get rid of jaundice. Water supplements do not lower the level of bilirubin in the blood. Some studies suggest water supplements are associated with higher bilirubin levels. Moreover, babies who are routinely given water tend to be nursed less frequently, and they have a higher rate of early weaning.

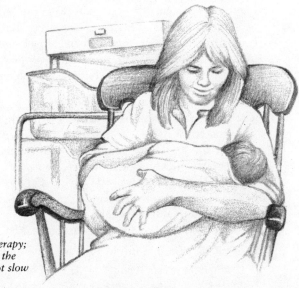

*Nurse often during phototherapy; taking the baby from under the bili-light for feedings will not slow her recovery from jaundice.*

**Treatment measures for jaundice**

1. Let the baby's physician know you prefer to continue nursing throughout the period of jaundice.
2. Nurse frequently, ideally every two to two and a half hours, and encourage the baby to suck at least 15 to 20 minutes at each breast. Taking the baby from under the bili-light for these feedings will not delay the effectiveness of treatment. Intermittent phototherapy is thought to be as effective as continuous exposure.
3. If your baby is sleepy, as jaundiced babies sometimes are, see Sleepy Baby.
4. Avoid water supplements, as these do not reduce bilirubin levels and may discourage the baby to nurse frequently.
5. If you are still hospitalized or you are welcome to stay in a room while your baby is being treated, ask the nurses if you can have the baby's crib and light set up next to your bed so you can care for the baby and nurse frequently.
6. If you cannot stay 24 hours a day with your baby, manually express or pump your milk every three hours (see Chapter 5). Take your milk to the hospital for the feedings you will miss.
7. If your doctor is firm in his or her desire for you to temporarily stop nursing, again, express or pump milk every three hours to keep your supply up. Freeze your milk and save it for later. In this case an electric pump is strongly recommended (see Appendix A).

## Difficult Latch-on: Refusal to Nurse

Latch-on problems can originate with the baby or the mother. Most occur when the baby is sleepy (see Sleepy Baby); when the breast becomes overly full or engorged (see Engorged Breasts); or when the mother has flat, dimpled, or inverted nipples (see Difficult Latch-on: Flat, Dimpled, or Inverted Nipples). Problems other than these are discussed as follows.

**The baby who has nursed earlier.** During the first week, it is not uncommon for a baby who has already nursed to suddenly refuse one or both sides. He may simply act uninterested although he is awake, or he may protest furiously when put to one or both breasts. A baby who has been given a bottle or pacifier during the first week may become "nipple confused" and refuse to nurse thereafter. Such a baby will likely start nursing again after a few hours uncoaxed or after one or more of the following measures are taken.

**Treatment measures for the baby who stops nursing**

1. Soften the areola if you are overly full or engorged by using manual expression or a pump just before putting the baby to breast.
2. Calm the frantic baby. A few drops of colostrum or glucose water on his

lips or dripped over the nipple will often alert and encourage him. Occasionally a very upset baby may need to be tightly swaddled in a thin blanket.

3. Pay attention to proper positioning (see Chapter 2). When the baby turns his face from side to side with mouth wide open, pull him in closer so his tongue can feel the nipple.

4. Try letting the baby suck on your finger for a few seconds just before putting him to breast.

5. If the baby seems to spit out the nipple with his tongue, try holding some ice against the nipple for a few minutes to firm it. This can be particularly effective for the baby who acts "nipple confused."

6. Persist. The baby who is hiccoughing, having a bowel movement, or staring at his mother or something else interesting will usually be reluctant to latch on. Try again in a half-hour or so.

7. Coax the baby who is suddenly refusing one breast by using the football hold on that side.

**The baby who has not yet nursed.** If a day or more has passed since the baby's birth and she still has not managed to latch on and suck, she probably has one of the specific problems described as follows.

*Tongue-tied.* Some of the infants in this situation are tongue-tied. The frenulum, or string-like tissue that attaches to the underside of the tongue, is so short or connected so close to the tip of the tongue that the baby may not be able to extend her tongue past her bottom lip. Although she can suck on a finger or rubber nipple that extends well into her mouth, she may be unable to grasp the underside of her mother's nipple. Occasionally, a tongue-tied baby can manage to latch onto one breast but not the other.

The solution is simple: the frenulum should be clipped to release

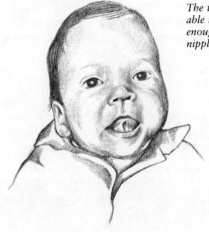

*The tongue-tied baby may not be able to extend his tongue far enough to latch on to his mother's nipple.*

the tongue. Some physicians are reluctant or unwilling to perform this procedure, however, since studies made several years ago showed that tongue-tied infants rarely develop speech difficulties later in life; the studies concluded that tongue clipping was therefore unnecessary. Unfortunately, though, some tongue-tied babies are unable to breastfeed. If you cannot persuade your doctor to clip the frenulum, find another who will. An experienced surgeon or dentist may do this in his or her office. The procedure takes just a minute.

*Tongue thrusting (nipple confusion).* Some babies push their tongues forward while trying to latch on or suck, and by doing so they spit the nipple out. Babies may do this from birth or as a result of sucking on a rubber nipple. When a rubber nipple is to blame, the problem is referred to as nipple confusion. Tongue-thrusting babies can usually relearn to nurse, with some assistance.

*Protruding tongue.* A few babies have tongues that protrude. The tongue sometimes looks longer than normal; it may be visible between the lips much of the time. Some mothers have described the tongue as forming a hump in the mouth that the nipple is not able to get past.

You may be able to teach the baby to nurse by encouraging her to open wide with her tongue down and pulling back behind the areola just before latch-on. The football hold is recommended for the best visibility and control. If you manage to get the baby on the breast, be sure she is sucking adequately. This means she does not come off the breast easily; is making long, drawing sucks; and is audibly swallowing. A few babies suck with the nipple in the front of the mouth; they rarely swallow and get very little milk.

*Tongue sucking.* Other infants who have difficulty latching on to the breast are those who suck their own tongues. These babies usually slide off the nipple after one or two sucks, and their cheeks dimple with each suck. They may also make clicking noises. When the baby opens her mouth to root or to cry, you may notice that her tongue is far back in her mouth or is curled toward the roof of her mouth.

Attempt to get the baby to latch on only when she opens wide with her tongue down. Stimulating the lower lip or slightly depressing the chin may help the tongue to drop. Pull the baby in very close. The football hold is best when you are working alone, and side-lying will give more control and visibility when someone is assisting you.

**When refusal persists.** If you have followed the preceding suggestions for a day or two and your baby still has not latched on, try the following measures.

**Treatment measures for refusal to nurse**

1. Continue working with the baby. Short, frequent sessions may be less upsetting for both of you. If someone is working with you, the side-lying position may give her the greatest control and visibility. These sessions can become intense and sometimes upsetting, so let your helper know if you or the baby needs a break. If you are in the hospital, let several nurses work with you; you may find one or two who are exceptionally skilled and sensitive.

2. Refuse any offers from nurses of rubber nipple shields or bottle nipples to place over your own nipple for nursing. Your baby will latch on and suck, but the shield does not allow for adequate nipple stimulation or for the necessary compression of the sinuses beneath the areola. This can seriously hamper the let-down of milk and adequate emptying of the breast, which may lead to a poor milk supply and insufficient intake for the baby. In addition, most babies will refuse ever to nurse without the shield.

3. If after 24 to 48 hours your baby has not latched on, supplementary feedings should begin. Manually express or pump your milk at least eight times a day, and feed the baby using an orthodontic shaped nipple (available at most drugstores). Many lactation professionals and mothers have found this type of nipple helpful in correcting latch-on problems.

4. If you are discharged from the hospital and your baby is still not nursing, locate an electric pump (see Appendix A) and keep giving your milk to the baby, using the orthodontic shaped nipple (see Chapter 3 for guidelines on pumping).

5. Continue short practice sessions several times a day. Some babies do better on a soft or empty breast.

6. Get lots of support and encouragement. If possible, see a lactation professional.

7. Be patient and persistent. Many babies with latch-on problems do overcome them sometime during the first ten days, but a significant number first latch on at about one month of age.

*Orthodontic nipples, such as the Nuk nipple, are best for bottle feeding.*

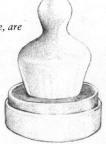

## Sucking Problems

Some babies latch on to the breast without difficulty but have a faulty sucking pattern. The suction is so poor that they easily slide off the breast or can be taken off effortlessly. When they are nursing their cheeks dimple with each suck, and you may hear frequent clicking noises. Most of these babies are sucking on their tongues and not on the nipple. It is thought that such infants suck on their tongues while in the uterus, and are born with this habit. They receive only the milk that drips into their mouths.

Although most babies with this problem have it from birth, others may develop it if they lose much weight, usually close to a pound, by the end of the first week. If this happens, and the baby cannot correct his suck after several good attempts at latching on, pump your milk and bottle-feed for 24 to 72 hours, supplementing breast milk with formula as necessary. After the baby is rehydrated and has regained a few ounces, he will probably correct his suck on his own.

A baby may have difficulty sucking at one or both breasts because she is tongue-tied. No matter how hard she tries, she may fail to get milk from the breast, and the mother's nipples may hurt even when the baby is correctly positioned. Sometimes a clicking sound can be heard as the baby sucks. To correct such a problem have your doctor or dentist clip the baby's frenulum. (See the section on tongue-tied babies under Difficult Latch-On: Refusal to Nurse.)

If your baby is born with a faulty suckling pattern but doesn't seem to be tongue-tied, follow the measures outlined as follows.

**Treatment measures for the baby who has a sucking problem from birth**

1. Remove the baby from the breast as soon as this pattern is evident.
2. Observe the position of the tongue when the baby's mouth is wide open. If it is curled against the roof of the mouth, try to lower it with your finger. Sometimes touching the lower lip or pressing slightly on the chin will help.
3. Using the football hold, pull the baby in as close as possible for latch-on.
4. Continue working with the baby. Short, frequent sessions may be less upsetting for both of you. If someone is working with you, the side-lying position may give her the greatest control and visibility. These sessions can become intense and upsetting, so let your helper know if you or the baby needs a break. If you are in the hospital, several nurses work with you; you may find one or two who are exceptionally skilled and sensitive.
5. Refuse any offers from nurses of rubber nipple shields or bottle nipples to place over your own nipple for nursing. Your baby will latch on and suck, but the shield does not allow for adequate nipple stimulation or for the necessary compression of the sinuses beneath the areola. This can seriously hamper the let-down of milk and adequate emptying of the breast,

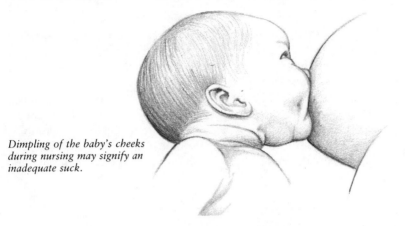

*Dimpling of the baby's cheeks during nursing may signify an inadequate suck.*

which may lead to a poor milk supply and insufficient intake for the baby. In addition, most babies will refuse ever to nurse without the shield.

6. If after 24 to 48 hours your baby still has not latched on, supplementary feedings should begin. Manually express or pump your milk at least eight times a day, and feed the baby using an orthodontic shaped nipple (available in most drugstores). Many experienced lactation professionals and mothers have found this type of nipple helpful in correcting sucking problems.

7. If you are discharged from the hospital and your baby still is not nursing, locate an electric pump (see Appendix A) and keep giving your milk to the baby, using an orthodontic shaped nipple (see Chapter 3 for guidelines on pumping).

8. Continue short practice sessions several times a day. Some babies do better on a soft or empty breast.

9. Get lots of support and encouragement. If possible, see a lactation professional.

10. Be patient and persist. Many babies with sucking problems do overcome them sometime during the first ten days, but a significant number first latch on at about one month of age.

## Fussiness and Excessive Night Waking

It can come as a surprise when your baby suddenly becomes fussy after spending most of his first few days sleeping. It is difficult to listen to your baby's cry; it may feel like an alarm going off in your body. Sometimes parents are told it is healthy for babies to cry, or that they will become spoiled if tended to every time they fuss. Comforting your infant and responding to her needs is very important to her well-being and her development of trust. Babies are really unspoilable.

Newborns cry for a variety of reasons. Often they are fussy their first night home from the hospital. They may be hungry as often as every hour, especially when the milk is just starting to come in, or when feedings have been limited because of their sleepiness or for other reasons. Some babies seem to need more sucking time than others. Some seem to pass a lot of gas, which causes them discomfort. Many newborns become upset when they are not kept snugly wrapped. Perhaps they miss the close, secure feeling of the womb.

Then there are the babies who sleep most of the day and wake frequently during the night. These babies are said to have their days and nights "mixed up."

### Coping measures for fussiness

1. Nurse your baby on demand, or at least every two to three hours for at least 15 to 20 minutes at each breast. If your nipples are sore and you are limiting feedings to 10 minutes per side, you may want to hold the baby and offer an orthodontic shaped pacifier after feedings.
2. Massage your breasts while you nurse to encourage the milk to let down.
3. Switch the baby back and forth between breasts several times during the feeding.
4. Burp the baby after she finishes at each breast. This will help prevent swallowed air from passing through the intestines and encourage her to nurse longer. If your baby is passing a lot of gas, you may need to burp her several times during each feeding. See Chapter 2 if you are having difficulty burping the baby.
5. Burp your baby after she uses a pacifier. Avoid using "stuffed" bottle nipples as pacifiers as these cause excessive air swallowing.
6. Wrap the baby snugly in a light blanket after feeding.
7. Avoid water or formula supplements. Perhaps you have nursed your baby but she acts as if she is still hungry. You can, certainly, offer her the breast again. But often newborn babies will stay awake after a feeding and behave as if they need to suck longer even though their bellies are full. Reassure yourself if needed, by referring to Underfeeding and Weight Loss. Most young infants will take additional water or formula if it is offered, even when they have had enough to eat, but this often leads to problems.

If your baby does not seem content after nursing, feel free to nurse her some more, or try comforting her next to your body. Rocking or walking with the baby for a while will usually keep her content. In an hour or two you can nurse her again.

### Coping measures for excessive night waking

1. Nurse your baby every two to two and a half hours during the daytime and evening. If the baby is sleeping through feeding times, see Sleepy Baby.
2. Tuck your baby in with you for a few nights; she may sleep better.

## Underfeeding and Weight Loss

During the first week, you may wonder if your baby is getting enough to eat. You may worry about whether the milk supply is adequate—especially when the baby seems to be nursing all the time or is fussy after feedings. Some mothers question whether they have milk when they observe the normal softening of the breast that occurs after the initial engorgement is gone. Weighing the baby will probably not provide reassurance, because newborns normally lose 5 to 10 percent of their birth weight during the first week, and most take two weeks to regain it.

Most newborns want to nurse 8 to 15 times in a 24-hour period after the first three to four days of life. This frequent nursing is normal and seldom reflects a poor milk supply or "weak milk." The baby is probably getting enough milk if—

- He is nursing at least eight times in 24 hours.
- You can hear him swallowing while nursing (when the room is quiet).
- Your breasts seem to soften somewhat after nursing.
- The number of wet diapers is starting to increase by the fourth or fifth day, or there are at least eight wet diapers in a 24-hour period after the fifth day.
- The baby is having yellow stools or frequent dark stools, or the stools are beginning to lighten in color by the fourth or fifth day.

Seeing if the baby will take a supplemental bottle of water or formula after nursing is not a reliable method of determining if he is getting enough breast milk. Most babies will take a few ounces if it is offered, even when they have had enough milk from the breasts. If your baby seems fussy and acts hungry after nursing, see Fussiness and Excessive Night Waking.

Excessive weight loss can occur when nursing is infrequent, when a mother is using a rubber nipple shield while nursing, when a baby has a faulty suck, or when a newborn is sick. Some stool softeners and laxatives, when taken by the mother, can cause a baby to have excessive bowel movements and to lose weight or to gain too slowly. Signs that a baby may not be receiving enough milk usually include all or most of the following:

- The baby is nursing six times or fewer in a 24-hour period after the third or fourth day after birth.
- The baby rarely swallows.
- The breasts do not soften after nursing.

- The baby is fussy or lethargic most of the time.
- The baby has dimples in his cheeks or makes clicking noises while nursing, and does not have good suction.
- The baby is wetting fewer than six diapers in a 24-hour period after the fifth day after birth.
- The baby is not having bowel movements at least once a day or is having small, dark stools after the fifth day after birth.

If your baby exhibits all or most of these signs, notify your doctor and have the baby weighed and examined. If you find that the baby has lost more than 10 percent of his birth weight, or very close to a pound, you and your doctor will need to decide on a course of action. Supplemental feeding may be necessary, but there are several ways to do this and still continue to nurse. If possible, see a lactation professional.

### Treatment measures for underfeeding

1. Be sure to nurse your baby at least ten times in every 24 hours. If the baby has an adequate suck, you might consider obtaining a nursing supplementation device (see Appendix A). In this way the baby can breastfeed and receive supplementary nutriments at the same time. This will increase both the baby's weight and your milk supply. Usually the device is needed for only a short time.
2. You may also increase your milk supply quickly by pumping your breasts after nursing (again, be sure you are nursing at least eight times in every 24 hours). An electric pump may be most efficient and convenient for this (see Appendix A). Feed your breast milk to the baby along with any necessary supplement; as soon as the baby's weight has increased, gradually stop supplementing.
3. If your baby has a sucking problem, pump your breasts at least eight times in every 24 hours and offer your milk by bottle along with any necessary supplement. An electric pump may be most efficient and convenient. See Sucking Problems for further help.

**If treatment fails.** It is frightening to suddenly realize that your new baby has lost an excessive amount of weight. Although the techniques just outlined will normally reverse the situation within several days, occasionally they won't work. Usually the underlying cause is the baby's faulty suck or a poor nursing pattern.

In unusual instances, a mother fails to produce milk. This sometimes happens to women who have had certain types of breast surgery (see Nursing after Breast Surgery, Chapter 3). Another group of women who cannot produce milk are those with insufficient glandular tissue. These women experience no breast enlargement during pregnancy, often have one breast that is significantly smaller than the other, and experience no fullness on the third to fifth day after birth (see Chapter 3).

In any of these situations, lack of support from family, friends, and professionals can only make matters worse. Even with all of the best information and support, things sometimes don't turn out as we hope. If you have given it your best but finally end up having to bottle-feed, you have not failed as a mother. Be proud of your efforts to nurse, and concentrate on providing your baby with all the cuddling and loving that you can.

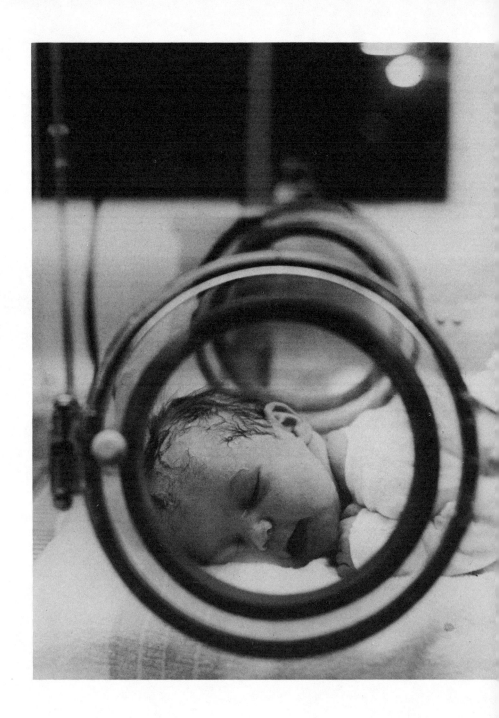

CHAPTER THREE

# Special Mothers, Special Babies

## Special Mothers

Medical Reasons for Not Breastfeeding
Medications and Environmental Pollutants
Nursing after Breast Surgery
Nursing an Adopted Baby
Relactation
The Diabetic Mother
The Mother with Herpes
The Epileptic Mother
Nursing and Thyroid Conditions

## Special Babies

The Premature Baby
Twins
The Baby with a Birth Defect
Developmental and Neurological Problems

NURSING CAN BE A SPECIAL CHALLENGE IN CERTAIN CIRCUMSTANCES—
circumstances that may result from a longstanding condition or that
may take you completely by surprise. Either way, you may be tempted
to give up the idea of breastfeeding altogether. The specific guidelines
in this chapter should help you make a realistic appraisal of your situation and find, I hope, the happiest solution for you and your baby.

# Special Mothers

## Medical Reasons for Not Breastfeeding

Occasionally a mother may have a medical or physical condition that
prevents her from breastfeeding. While most medical conditions a
mother might have pose no harm to her nursing infant, a few are reasons not to breastfeed.

A mother with active tuberculosis should not breastfeed until treatment has been administered for one to three weeks, when she can no
longer transmit the infection.

Lumps in the breast are common. Even if a lump needs to be surgically removed, weaning is not necessary. But a mother who is diagnosed with breast cancer should forego nursing so she may undertake
immediate treatment.

In the case of a mother with hepatitis B, the American Academy of
Pediatrics feels that the risk of transmission to the infant is very low.
The mother should breastfeed provided her baby is immunized against
the virus immediately after birth.

Mothers infected with AIDS (Acquired Immune Deficiency Syndrome) are discouraged from breastfeeding until more is known about
the transmission of the virus.

Although the overwhelming majority of women can produce a full
supply of milk for their infants, even after a setback due to infrequent
nursing or inadequate sucking (see Survival Guide for the First Week),
a few mothers are unable to produce enough milk. A low milk supply
can occur when a mother has had extensive breast surgery (see Nursing after Breast Surgery). A relatively uncommon condition is that of
insufficient glandular tissue. In this case a mother finds that her
breasts did not enlarge during pregnancy and did not undergo *any*
changes (such as heaviness, fullness, or leaking of milk) during the
first week after delivery. Most often the mother has one breast that is
significantly smaller than the other. In this case she can still nurse her
baby by using a nursing supplementation device designed to provide
the extra milk needed (see Appendix A).

## Medications and Environmental Pollutants

A mother may occasionally wonder if her milk is entirely safe for her child. Most frequently, this concern arises because she needs to take medication. Although most medications pass into the breast milk, the majority are considered safe for the nursing infant. A comprehensive guide to drugs in breast milk can be found in Appendix B.

More and more questions have arisen about the environmental pollutants we are exposed to, such as insecticides and other toxic chemicals. Many of these substances are stored in fatty tissues of the body, and, as a result, small amounts may be detected in breast milk. Experts on the subject, however, have been unable to identify any risks to the baby from such amounts, and most believe that the nutritional and immunological benefits of breast milk far outweigh the possible risks of environmental pollutants. Sadly, our children receive even greater exposure to some of these chemicals in the womb than they do at the breast.

Some women have been exposed to high concentrations of polychlorinated biphenyl (PCB) or polybrominated biphenyl (PBB), both toxic chemicals. Mothers who for many years have eaten more than one meal a week of sport-caught fish from the Great Lakes or certain of its tributaries, who live on PCB-silo farms, or who have been employed for years handling PCB, should consider having their milk tested for this toxin. Information about analyzing breast milk can be obtained from state health department laboratories. PBB is less frequently found in the food chain; however, it was accidentally added to cattle feed in Michigan during 1973. Mothers in Michigan's general population were subsequently found to have low levels of PBB in their breast milk—levels determined to pose no threat to nursing infants. Women on quarantined farms had higher levels, but their children, many of whom were breastfed, showed no signs of illness or any effect on their growth and development.

Nursing mothers who want to reduce their exposure to toxic chemicals should certainly stop using pesticides in the home, avoid eating fish caught in contaminated waters, stay away from permanently moth-proofed garments, carefully wash or peel fresh fruits and vegetables, and avoid crash diets, which are likely to increase the excretion of toxic substances into breast milk.

Processed infant formulas are not without their own potential hazards. Besides lacking the immunological properties of breast milk that keep the infant healthy, they can easily become contaminated when the person preparing the baby's bottle does not take proper care in handling and storing the formula and equipment. Parents frequently don't pay close attention when diluting powdered and liquid formula concentrates. From time to time too, manufacturing errors in the production of infant formulas have had serious consequences. High levels of aluminum have been identified in most formulas (Weintraub et al., 1986).

## Nursing After Breast Surgery

When performed prior to a woman's giving birth, minor breast surgery such as a biopsy or removal of a lump seldom affects the woman's ability to nurse. A woman who has undergone a mastectomy can nurse on the remaining breast, and by nursing frequently she can usually provide all the milk her baby needs.

When a surgical implantation has been performed to alter the size and shape of the breasts, milk production is usually not affected unless the milk ducts have been severed (this may be the case if the incision was made along the edge of the areola). In the case of a breast reduction, milk production depends on the amount of breast tissue removed and the extensiveness of the surgery. When the nipples have been relocated on the breast the ducts have usually been severed, and so the milk supply is often deficient. Some mothers have continued breastfeeding with the aid of a nursing supplementation device when their milk supply has proven to be insufficient as a result of previous breast surgery (see Appendix A).

## Nursing an Adopted Baby

More and more mothers who are planning to adopt babies are considering breastfeeding them. An infant's suck can stimulate milk production whether or not the mother has ever had or nursed a baby before. Most adoptive mothers, however, need to supplement their breast milk, many for the entire time they are nursing. Probably the safest and most convenient way to supplement breastfeeding is with a nursing supplementation device, which is specifically designed for this situation (see Appendix A).

It is impossible to predict whether an adoptive mother will be able to produce milk, or how much she will produce, even if she is currently nursing or has recently nursed another baby. Adoptive nursing will be most successful if you focus on the baby and your relationship rather than on milk production. Measure your success by whether the experience truly helps make the baby yours.

Before the baby arrives, it is wise to learn as much as possible about breastfeeding and adoptive nursing. Be sure to talk with a pediatrician

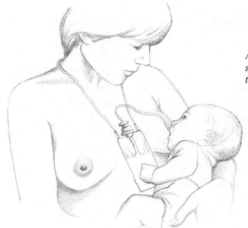

*As the baby nurses,*
*she can get immediate satisfaction*
*through a supplementation device.*

who will be supportive of your efforts. A lactation professional may be able to refer you to other adoptive mothers who have nursed their babies. Several publications are also available on nursing adoptive babies; they are listed in Appendix A.

You may be told you should try to initiate milk production before the baby's arrival by expressing or pumping the breasts several times a day. There is debate over whether this is beneficial over the long run.

You may be hoping for donations of breast milk to use in the supplementation device, and perhaps you've already received offers of donated milk. But don't expect others to continue donations indefinitely. It can be a real effort for nursing mothers to collect extra milk. There is also a remote possibility that an infectious disease could be transmitted through donated milk.

Your baby may be easily persuaded to begin nursing, or she may require a great deal of patience and persistence. It has been generally found that the younger the baby, the easier the transition from the bottle to the breast. See the Survival Guide for the First Week for assistance in getting the baby to nurse.

## Relactation

For a variety of reasons, a mother may want to begin nursing after starting her baby on the bottle, or to resume nursing after weaning her baby.

If your baby has never nursed but is less than a week old, or if less than a week has passed since you weaned, nursing every two hours will usually stimulate full milk production within a few days. This is true even if you have taken medication to "dry up" your milk. To speed relactation, switch the baby back and forth from one breast to the other during nursings. You may need to supplement your milk for a few days with small amounts of formula or donated breast milk; offer the supplement *after* nursing the baby. It is important that the baby be carefully monitored to be sure he is getting enough to eat during this period of transition.

If the baby has never been nursed and is older than a week, or if a week or more has passed since weaning, frequent nursing with supplementation is necessary during the period of relactation. A nursing supplementation device is generally recommended for both safety and convenience. The baby in this situation, like the adopted baby, may require weeks or months of supplementation, depending on the length of time since delivery or weaning.

## The Diabetic Mother

Many diabetic mothers enjoy the advantages of nursing. For them breastfeeding often stimulates a remission-like response, resulting in a decreased need for insulin and an increased need for calories. Babies of diabetic mothers are less likely to develop the disease themselves later in life if they are breastfed rather than formula-fed.

If you are diabetic, your requirements for insulin and calories will need to be closely monitored—especially during the early hours after delivery, when your insulin needs will drop dramatically.

For the first day or two, your newborn's blood sugar must be closely watched as her body adjusts to receiving less glucose than it did during pregnancy. She may need frequent nursing, and possibly supplemental glucose by nipple or IV, until her glucose levels stabilize. Because the infant of the diabetic mother is commonly delivered a few weeks early, she may also have respiratory problems and is more prone to becoming jaundiced.

Throughout the months of breastfeeding, careful monitoring of your glucose level, insulin dose, and caloric requirements must continue. As the baby stimulates increased milk production, you and your doctor will need to adjust your insulin dosage and caloric intake to prevent insulin reactions.

You should take particular care to avoid sore nipples and breast infections. This means giving careful attention to correct positioning of the baby, watching for signs of thrush (yeast) in the baby's mouth and on the nipples (see the Survival Guide for the First Week), and getting plenty of rest. Yeast infections are very common in the diabetic mother and her infant. Plugged ducts and other early signs of breast infection (see the Survival Guide for the First Two Months) should be treated promptly.

When weaning begins and milk production declines, you'll need to readjust your insulin dosage and diet again. This will be easier if you wean the baby slowly.

## The Mother with Herpes

If you have an active genital herpes lesion or a positive culture near your due date, and you therefore deliver by cesarean, you will most likely be given a private room. So long as the lesion is well covered and you wash your hands thoroughly before feedings, you can nurse the baby safely without gloves. When you are feeling better, there is no reason that you cannot share a room with the baby as long as you maintain these basic precautions. Should you have a herpes outbreak at home, the same principles apply.

Herpes Type I lesions are generally those that develop above the waist, usually on the mouth. Frequently they appear as cold sores or fever blisters. It is important for you, or any other person with an active lesion, to wash your hands thoroughly before touching the baby and, of course, avoid placing him in contact with the sores.

Occasionally a mother will develop a herpes lesion on her breast, nipple, or areola. Should you have such an outbreak, express or pump your milk until the lesion is gone.

## The Epileptic Mother

Most medications to control the occurrence of epileptic seizures are considered safe for nursing; however, it is best to check out any drug with your doctor. Major anticonvulsant medications are listed in Appendix B, where their safety is discussed.

A nursing mother with epilepsy offers these suggestions for others (Brewster, 1979):

- Have cribs or playpens available in various areas of the house; place gates across stairways and doorways.
- Nurse in a large upholstered chair, or pad the arms of a rocking chair.
- Use guard rails and pillows around the bed for night nursing.
- When alone on outings with the baby, tag the stroller or carrier with the name of the baby and the name of a person to contact in the event that you have a seizure.

*Nursing and Thyroid Conditions*

**Hypothyroidism.** Symptoms of an underactive thyroid gland may include extreme fatigue, poor appetite, and sometimes a low milk supply. Thyroid replacement quickly reverses these symptoms. The mother who is taking medication for hypothyroidism can breastfeed, as these drugs do not affect the baby.

**Hyperthyroidism.** Occasionally a doctor will discover that a nursing mother has an enlarged thyroid gland. Signs of hyperthyroidism include weight loss, increased appetite, nervousness, rapid heart rate, and palpitations. Nursing must be discontinued for at least 48 hours when radioactive iodine is used for diagnostic testing; however, other tests are available that do not require this interruption. If radioactive iodine is used, express or pump your milk and dispose of it.

If you are taking medication for an overactive thyroid gland, you can breastfeed as long as the specific medication is considered safe for the nursing baby. PTU (propylthiouracil) is the drug of choice, since it has the least effect on a baby's thyroid gland. The baby's thyroid level should be closely monitored. If necessary, the pediatrician can order thyroid replacement.

# Special Babies

## The Premature Baby

The days after giving birth to a premature baby can be overwhelming, particularly if the baby is sick or very immature. The mother of a premie may have doubts about many things, including her ability to nurse the baby.

If your baby is premature, it is especially important that he receive your milk. Your milk is particularly suited for his special growth needs and is easier for him to digest than formula. Premature infants are at greater risk for developing infections and are less able to cope with them, should they arise. The antibodies in your milk will provide your baby with protection against many of these infections. By providing breast milk, many mothers of premature infants have felt that they were able to contribute something special to their baby's well-being.

If your baby is three to five weeks early, you may be able to begin breastfeeding right away. The sick or very small premie may be unable to nurse for a while, but you can express your milk for him until he is well or mature enough to begin nursing. In this way he can still receive your milk, and you will have established your milk supply by the time he is ready to begin breastfeeding.

**Expressing milk for your baby.** If your baby is unable to nurse, start expressing your colostrum as soon after delivery as possible. Colostrum is especially beneficial for him as it is highly concentrated with protective antibodies. The nursing staff should provide you with a suitable pump and instructions for collecting and storing your milk. Many maternity units have an electric breast pump available. A fully automatic electric breast pump is most suited for a mother who is pumping around the clock for a premie (see Appendix A). If your baby is being transferred to another hospital for care, ask the transport team about their procedures for collecting, storing, and transporting your milk. If you will be following the baby to a special care nursery in another city, try to get a pump to take along with you.

You may receive differing bits of advice on how often and how long to pump your breasts. Keep in mind that your supply of milk depends on the frequent stimulation of your breasts. You should plan on expressing milk as often as your baby would nurse or at least eight times in 24 hours. Many nursery staffs suggest that women pump every three to four hours during the day and sleep all night. With this limited stimulation, most mothers find that after a while their milk supply dwindles. Determine a reasonable schedule for yourself that includes

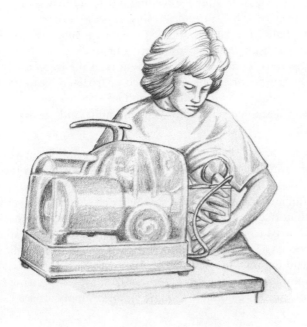

eight pumpings in 24 hours. Some mothers prefer to express their milk every three hours around the clock, whereas others would rather pump more often during the day so they can sleep for longer periods at night.

When you first begin to express milk you will probably start out getting just a few drops of colostrum. Until your milk is in, pump each breast for about five minutes, then return to each breast a second time for a few more minutes.

After your milk is in, pump each breast until the flow subsides. Return to each breast a second or third time for a few more minutes. Gently massaging each breast for a minute or so before you begin and while you are pumping will help your milk to let down. The whole process should take no more than 20 to 30 minutes.

Special care must be taken when expressing and storing your milk. Be sure to wash your hands before handling your breasts or any of the pump equipment. All pump parts that come in contact with the milk or your breasts must be thoroughly scrubbed with hot soapy water after each use and sterilized in boiling water or a dishwasher twice a day. Your daily bath or shower will cleanse your breasts sufficiently.

After collecting your milk, pour it into a sterile container, according to your nursery staff's preference. Check with your baby's nurses on how much to put in each container to avoid wasting milk. Milk cannot be refrozen or refrigerated after it has been thawed or warmed; whatever is left over after the feeding must be thrown out.

Whenever possible, provide freshly expressed or refrigerated milk for your baby. Freezing the milk preserves many, but not all, of its protective substances. You can keep your milk for 24 to 48 hours in the refrigerator or for up to three months in the freezer.

When transporting your refrigerated or frozen milk to the hospital, pack the containers in ice inside a small ice chest or cooler. Some families use refreezable ice packs to keep the milk cold, or dry ice to keep it frozen.

*Expressing milk longer than two weeks.* Depending on your baby's maturity and general progress, you may find yourself expressing milk for a while. It is important that you eat well, get plenty to drink, and rest enough to maintain your own energy as well as your milk supply.

If you notice that your milk supply is declining a few days in a row, you will need to assess the situation and make whatever adjustments are necessary. The most common cause of a decreasing milk supply is infrequent expression—fewer than eight times in 24 hours. Although a few mothers can maintain a good milk supply expressing less often than this, most are not able to keep up their supply after a few weeks.

If you have been using a hand pump, you may want to consider renting an electric pump. Most mothers find an electric pump requires less effort and is generally more efficient and convenient.

Besides increasing the number of pumpings per day, switch from one breast to the other several times as soon as you notice the flow slowing down. This technique is very effective for increasing milk production. Pumping both breasts simultaneously, using one of the double collection kits manufactured by the makers of electric breast pumps, is also a very effective way to increase your milk production and decrease your pumping time. With these kits most mothers can express their milk in 10 to 15 minutes.

Occasionally you may notice that your milk supply drops when you and your baby have a difficult day. This is normal and usually temporary. Stress can temporarily decrease your milk supply. The following suggestions have proved helpful when this occurs:

- Pump regularly, every two to three hours.
- Take a short nap or a warm bath just before expressing.
- Apply moist heat to your breasts before expressing.
- Massage each breast as you are pumping, or stimulate the opposite nipple.
- Ask someone to rub your back between the shoulder blades while you are pumping.
- If possible, hold the baby while you are pumping at the hospital, or keep a photo of your baby with your pump.

If these measures do not help the milk to let down faster and more frequently, check with your doctor, who may prescribe oxytocin nasal spray. Refer to Let-down Problems in the Survival Guide for the First Week.

**When breastfeeding begins.** When the time arrives to begin nursing the premature infant, most mothers have very high expectations. Premies' abilities at the breast vary greatly, but most are unable to complete an entire feeding at first.

Have a nurse help you during the first few sessions. Your goal is to position the baby well for nursing and to encourage him to latch on to the nipple. These early practice sessions go best when the baby is awake and alert and the breast is not overly full. Keeping the baby wrapped in a blanket will usually discourage his interest. Most premies will stay warm undressed next to their mother's body. The nurse can check the baby's skin temperature after 5 to 10 minutes.

The football hold is the position of choice for nursing a premature baby. This hold offers the most visibility and control over the baby's

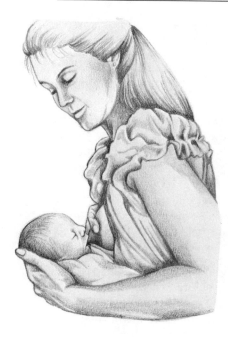

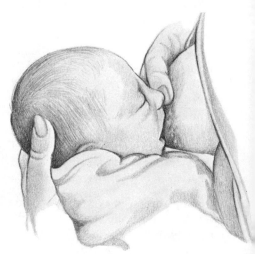

*Interesting a premie in nursing requires extra effort: use the football hold, and place the nipple in his mouth.*

position. Support your breast with all your fingers beneath it and only the thumb on top. Lightly stroke the baby's lips with the nipple to signal him to open wide. As soon as he does, pull his head in so close that the nipple is on top of his tongue.

Again, premies' abilities at the breast vary greatly, so be patient. As long as you have positioned him correctly and are encouraging him to open his mouth, you have been successful.

Once latched on to the breast and sucking, a premie may fall asleep after just a few minutes. He may need a supplement after nursing until he is feeding more vigorously at the breast. Some hospitals do not give nursing premies supplements by bottle, but most do. If your nursery routinely offers a bottle after nursing, request that the nurse use an orthodontic nipple to minimize your baby's confusion with your own nipple.

While you are nursing your baby, you should be able to hear him swallowing. This means he is sucking effectively and getting your milk. If you do not hear swallowing, make sure the baby is actually latched on to the breast. His suction should be so strong that it is hard to pull him off. You should not see dimples in his cheeks or hear clicking noises as he sucks. These signs usually indicate he is sucking on his tongue and not on your nipple.

When the baby seems interested in the second breast, you can simply pass his head and body over to the other side, or you can reposition him entirely in the opposite arm using the football hold.

To maintain your milk supply, be sure to pump after these feeding sessions with the baby.

*Difficult latch-on.* Many premature infants have difficulty latching on, due to their own immaturity as well as having received rubber nipples as pacifiers or for feedings. Some babies have trouble learning to lower their tongue to latch on, whereas others seem unable to identify their mother's nipples in their mouths.

If your baby has not been able to latch on to the breast, refer to Difficult Latch-on: Refusal to Nurse, in the Survival Guide for the First Week. In my experience, most premature infants learn to nurse after a period of daily practice sessions.

**The transition to full-time nursing.** While you and the baby are establishing nursing, you may wonder how much milk the baby is taking. This is best estimated by the length of time he sucks and swallows as well as the softness of your breasts after nursing. If you have been pumping for a while you should be able to judge this fairly well. Pumping just after nursing will also give you an idea how much milk has been taken. Weighing the baby before and after nursing is not a good idea, since the baby may empty his bladder or bowels between weighings and thus falsify the reading.

Until your baby is nursing without any supplemental feedings, you will need to continue expressing milk after each nursing to maintain your milk supply. When your baby is actively sucking and swallowing for at least 15 minutes at a time, you can probably give up supplemental feedings and pumpings. Periodically checking the baby's weight may help guide you as well.

## Twins

Needless to say, caring for two babies takes a tremendous amount of time and energy. Breastfeeding twins is not only more healthful and economical than giving them formula, but in many ways it is more convenient. So long as the babies are nursing frequently, the average mother will have an abundant supply of milk for each.

As soon as you become aware of the twins during pregnancy, you should begin some special preparations. You will want to arrange for as much help as possible, of course, for the first several weeks after the birth. It's also a good idea to get to know other mothers who have successfully nursed their twins. Many communities have organizations for mothers of twins. You might also contact your local breastfeeding support group; such a group usually provides literature on caring for and nursing twins.

Approximately half of all twins are born prematurely. During pregnancy you can do much to lessen the risk of premature delivery and other complications by maintaining a diet high in calories—at least 2,900 a day—and protein—at least 110 grams a day. Talk with your health care provider about monitoring yourself for signs of preterm labor.

**Breastfeeding two.** Some mothers prefer nursing their babies together as much as possible, whereas others choose to nurse them separately. Nursing both twins at once certainly saves time, and it may be necessary when both of the babies are hungry. If you want to nurse the babies together, there are three basic positions you can try:

- both babies in the cuddle hold with their legs side by side or crossed over each other,
- one baby in the cuddle hold and the other in the football hold, or
- both babies in the football hold.

During the early weeks, you may need assistance getting the babies on the breast at the same time. You will also probably need a few pillows for positioning. (A special pillow is available for nursing twins. See Appendix A for ordering information.) It may be easier to position the baby who nurses less vigorously first, and then put the vigorous nurser to the breast. Nursing the twins simultaneously should get easier as they get older and need less head support and assistance latching on.

Nursing the babies separately may be easier to manage and will allow you more time with each individually. You may decide to feed each baby whenever she seems hungry or you may prefer to encourage the babies to eat and sleep on a similar schedule. To maintain a similar routine for both babies, simply offer the breast to the second baby, waking him if necessary, after nursing the first. Although most twins eventually develop a preference for one breast over the other, it is wise to alternate the babies at each feeding during the early weeks so the breasts will be evenly stimulated; this is particularly important when one baby is more active than the other. Keeping a simple written record may be helpful at first. After the first few days you might instead try assigning one breast to each baby for the day, and then switching the babies the next day.

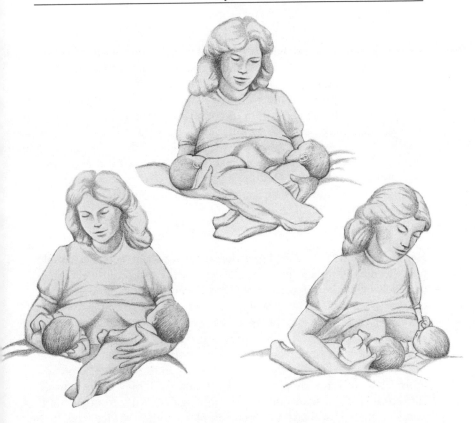

During the early weeks, bottle feeding is best avoided. You want to be sure your breasts are stimulated by the babies' sucking so that milk production remains adequate. Forgoing the bottle also helps to minimize the occurrence of plugged ducts and breast infections.

**Caring for yourself.** For the mother who is nursing twins, plenty of rest, food, and drink is essential. Most nursing mothers are naturally more hungry and thirsty, but if you take on too much and become fatigued, you may lose your appetite and too much weight. Nutritionists recommend that a mother nursing twins consume at least three thousand calories daily. Your diet should include high-protein foods and one to two quarts of milk a day, the equivalent in other dairy products, or a calcium supplement. Vitamin C and B-complex supplements may also be beneficial.

## The Baby with a Birth Defect

It may be that the baby with a birth defect needs her mother's milk, and the comfort and security of the breast, even more than other infants. Nursing such a baby is usually possible, but it is important that the mother is supported in her efforts. Although some mothers of babies with birth defects have been discouraged from attempting breastfeeding, many have gone on to nurse their babies successfully.

Depending on your baby's problem, you may be able to begin nursing right after birth, or you may need to express milk for a while (see Expressing Milk for Your Baby). Whatever the circumstances, it may be helpful to seek guidance from a breastfeeding counselor or another supportive professional. Some helpful publications are listed at the end of the book.

**Heart defect.** Infants with heart defects generally have little trouble breastfeeding. The exception is the baby with a severe defect, who may become easily fatigued or stressed during feedings; she will start breathing rapidly, her heart will beat faster, and her overall color may change. Her growth may be greatly affected due to the abnormality of her heart. She may also be more prone to infections, and therefore in greater need of breast milk than other babies.

The baby who becomes stressed during feedings needs to be nursed more frequently for shorter periods of time. She may also be more comfortable when held upright for nursing, as in the football hold. Some mothers have used a nursing supplementation device to reduce the baby's exertion at the breast (see Appendix A).

**Cleft lip and palate.** Breastfeeding a baby with a cleft lip, cleft palate, or both is rarely encouraged by medical professionals. It is sometimes possible, however, depending on the extent of the cleft. Feeding a baby with a cleft lip or palate by any method is difficult and time consuming, but nursing, when possible, is better for the baby because it requires full use of the facial muscles and thus promotes proper facial growth and development. Additionally, breast milk helps to reduce the number and severity of ear and respiratory infections, which are more common with these babies than others.

The baby born with a cleft lip alone may have little difficulty nursing. Until the lip is repaired, the baby needs to be positioned with the cleft sealed, to permit suction. You may insure a complete seal just by pulling the baby close against your breast, or you may need to place your finger or thumb over the cleft. If you find that your baby has more difficulty nursing on one side, it may help to use the football hold on that side.

Whether you can nurse a baby with a cleft palate usually depends on the location and extent of the cleft. When it is in the soft palate only, the baby may be able to nurse without much difficulty. It's best to position him so his head is raised; milk may come out of his nose if he is fed while lying flat. When the baby has an extensive cleft palate or cleft palate and lip, nursing can be difficult and is sometimes impossible. You will probably need to express milk for some time; eventually you may need to use formula, since a cleft palate is generally not repaired until the baby is several months old. Talk to the plastic surgeon about your desire to breastfeed.

Several techniques have been reported to help babies with cleft palates to breastfeed. An infant may be fitted with a plastic dental appliance that covers the cleft and allows for adequate sucking; ask your doctor about this possibility. Some lactation professionals have reported success with the use of a nursing supplementation device (see Appendix A).

Several mothers have described to me positioning techniques that have allowed their infants to nurse. If the nipple is angled away from the cleft, adequate suction may be achieved. An upright football hold may offer the best control over the baby's position. Some mothers have taught their babies to nurse by compressing the nipple behind the areola between the index and middle fingers, and holding it in the baby's mouth as far back as possible. Sources for additional information are listed at the end of the book.

## Developmental and Neurological Problems

Babies with Down's syndrome, hydrocephalus, spina bifida, and other neurological problems may benefit greatly from breastfeeding. Because nursing provides frequent physical contact, it may be especially valuable to such a baby's development.

If the baby's sucking ability is affected, teaching her to nurse will require a great deal of patience. Professional guidance from a lactation professional experienced with such problems and a physical therapist will probably be essential. When a baby is unable to suck, some mothers have been able to nurse with a nursing supplementation device (see Appendix A) or have provided their expressed milk in a bottle. Sources of additional information are listed at the end of the book.

**Down's syndrome.** Not only will nursing further the development of the infant with Down's syndrome, but it may also provide him with much needed protection from illness, as he is often at greater risk for developing infections than most babies. Although many infants with Down's syndrome are able to nurse, some have difficulty learning how to latch on and suck effectively. Frequently, the baby has weak muscle tone and may act sleepy and uninterested in the breast. He will need to be wakened or roused frequently for nursing (see Sleepy Baby, Survival Guide for the First Week).

Typically, the baby with Down's syndrome grows slowly. If his suck is weak and inefficient, a nursing supplementation device may be helpful in strengthening his sucking pattern and providing additional food.

**Hydrocephalus and spina bifida.** These birth defects are usually corrected surgically as soon as possible. Until the baby can begin to nurse, the mother must express milk (see Expressing Milk for Your Baby). For many such babies, positioning at the breast requires special attention so that they are protected and comfortable.

**Cerebral palsy.** Babies with cerebral palsy may also be able to nurse, depending on the severity of their conditions. Breastfeeding problems that occur are usually related to either (1) poor muscle tone and a weak suck or (2) excessive muscle tone (rigidity and abnormal posture), tongue thrusting, clenching of the jaw, and difficulty swallowing. Both of these situations usually lead to slow weight gain. Many infants with cerebral palsy are able to breastfeed successfully with a nursing supplementation device.

# CHAPTER FOUR

# The Learning Period: The First Two Months

## Now that You Are Postpartum

Caring for Yourself
Nutritional Needs

## Nursing Your Baby

Your Nursing Style
Your Milk Supply
Infant Dietary Supplements
Illnesses: Yours and the Baby's
The First Two Months: What's Normal?

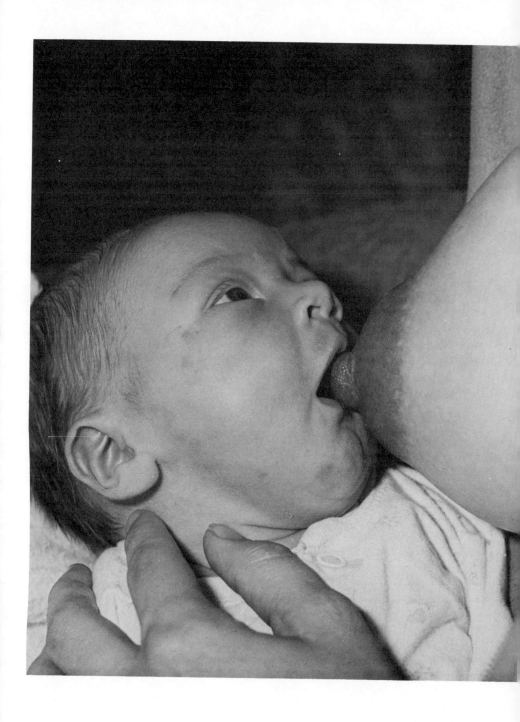

AFTER THE FIRST WEEK, YOU MAY ALREADY BE FEELING ENERGETIC and confident in your abilities as a new mother—or you may be exhausted, overwhelmed, and perhaps troubled with some aspect of breastfeeding. In any case, it is important to realize that the first two months after giving birth are a time for adjustment and learning. Mothers normally have questions and concerns about themselves, their babies, and nursing during this period.

# Now that You Are Postpartum

## *Caring for Yourself*

Postpartum is the six-week period in which all of the many changes of pregnancy are reversed. Virtually every system in your body will go through some readjustment. As your uterus shrinks in size and the inner lining is shed, a new layer is formed. The vaginal flow, or lochia, decreases in amount and progresses to pink or brown by the end of the first week and then to white by about the tenth day postpartum. Too much activity during the early weeks can cause the lochia to become heavier and return to pink or red—a signal to slow down.

If you have had a vaginal birth, your vagina, perineum, urethra, and rectum have undergone considerable stress. Frequent warm baths will speed healing and help relieve discomfort. Kegel's exercises will help this area return to normal by strengthening the entire pelvic floor. These exercises are simple and can be done anytime, anywhere. Several times a day, tightly squeeze the muscles around your anus, then around your vagina and urethra. Gradually work up to 100 "kegels" a day.

If you have had a cesarean birth, keep in mind you are recovering from major abdominal surgery. Most likely, you will still need to take pain medication during the first week or so at home. You may perhaps be bothered by an uncomfortable feeling that your abdomen may fall out. A lightweight girdle can provide some welcome support.

Constipation is a common complaint after giving birth. It can best be prevented by drinking plenty of fluids, adding fiber to your diet, and getting regular exercise. Be aware that some stool softeners and laxatives could affect the baby, causing cramping, excessive stools, and even weight loss.

Starting at approximately six to twelve weeks postpartum, some women experience generalized hair loss (telogeneffluvium). Because of the hormonal changes following birth, hair follicles simultaneously move from the growing phase (which they were in during pregnancy) to the resting phase of their development. Postpartum hair loss is seldom severe, and women never go bald because of it. The period of hair loss lasts about three to six months. It has no relationship to breastfeeding.

Most women experience emotional changes during the postpartum period. Anxiety, moodiness, and irritability are common responses to the hormonal changes that occur after giving birth, as well as to the tremendous responsibility of caring for a new baby. Some mothers notice other postpartum "symptoms" such as forgetfulness, inability to concentrate, and difficulty expressing thoughts. These problems seem to pass with time. If you fall prey, though, to exhaustion, poor nutrition, and isolation from other adults, depression may be the result.

Because of the rapid physical changes of the postpartum period and the tremendous amount of time and energy needed to care for and nurse a baby, rest should continue to take high priority for all new mothers. Lack of rest can slow your recovery from the birth and may lead to tension, inability to cope, poor appetite, and depression. Be

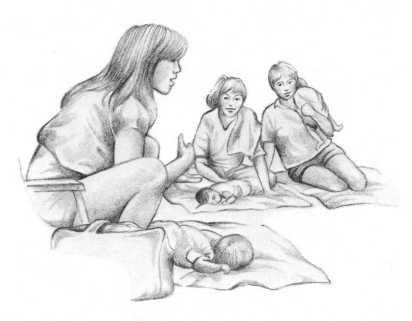

*New mothers' groups provide opportunities for socializing as well as learning about infant development.*

sure to take at least one nap every day during these important first weeks. Do essential household chores and activities while the baby is awake so that you can nap together. Tucking the baby in with you at nap time and bedtime may help you both sleep better. Getting plenty of rest now will contribute greatly to your sense of well-being and your breastfeeding success.

After a couple of weeks some light exercise can do much to renew your energy. A brisk twenty-minute walk with the baby can be invigorating; the fresh air will do you both good. Many community centers offer exercise programs for new mothers. The babies are often included in the exercises, or infant care may be provided. With whatever activity you choose, of course, you will want to start out slowly.

You may feel isolated as a new mother, especially if you have left work or school—and most of your friends—to care for the baby. You need adult companionship. Check with your childbirth educator or public health nurse about groups for new mothers. Attending La Leche League meetings, taking a mother-baby exercise class, or socializing with women from your childbirth class are excellent ways of getting out with the baby and getting to know other new mothers.

## Nutritional Needs

**Drinking enough.** Maintaining an adequate intake of fluids is usually not a problem for the nursing mother. Most women are naturally more thirsty while they are breastfeeding. Contrary to popular belief, forcing fluids beyond satisfying natural thirst does not increase milk production.

But when a nursing mother does not drink at least six to eight glasses of fluids every day, dark, concentrated urine and constipation usually result. She may need to make a conscious effort to increase her fluid intake.

**Eating well.** Provided you established good eating habits during pregnancy and gained an adequate amount of weight, you probably won't need to change your diet much at all. The ideal diet for a nursing mother provides about five hundred calories more than her pre-pregnancy diet, including 65 grams of protein. You can get the extra nutrients in between-meal snacks, perhaps during nursings: half a sandwich and a glass of milk, three glasses of juice, or two-thirds cup of peanuts will supply about five hundred calories. Some mothers experience a temporary loss of appetite the first couple of weeks after delivery. Eating smaller, more frequent meals or snacks may be more appealing.

You may feel discouraged that your shape is not back to normal. The clothes in your closet may seem as if they belonged to someone else. Although you lost some weight when you delivered, you are probably still pounds away from your usual weight. During the early months of breastfeeding, this extra fat is a useful energy store. If you let your appetite guide you as you continue nursing, you will probably lose the excess weight gradually and feel good while doing it. Dieting during the early weeks is not a good idea.

If you like, you can estimate your daily caloric needs by multiplying your current weight by 15. Add 500 to your total to meet the caloric needs of nursing (if you are nursing twins, add 1,000 calories). If you are a moderately active woman, you can expect to lose a pound every two to three weeks on this diet. If you are very active and have no problem controlling your weight, or if you burn calories slowly, you will need to adjust the figures somewhat: multiply your weight by 17 (high activity) or 13 (low activity).

$$
\begin{array}{r}
\textit{Example:} \quad 135 \text{ pounds} \\
\times 15 \\
\hline
2{,}025 \text{ calories} \\
+ \ 500 \text{ calories} \\
\hline
2{,}525 \text{ calories}
\end{array}
$$

Milk production is largely independent of nutritional intake during the first few months of breastfeeding. This is partly because the fat accumulated in pregnancy is available as a ready supply of calories. When a mother's diet is inadequate, however, milk production usually continues at her expense—leading to fatigue, listlessness, and rapid weight loss.

Some women have trouble finding time to fix nutritious meals for themselves when they are at home alone with the baby. If you find yourself in this situation, start the day with a good breakfast, and then snack throughout the day on nutritious foods such as hard-boiled eggs, leftover chicken or beef, cheese, peanut butter, yogurt, seeds, and nuts. Don't forget the fiber: whole-wheat bread, whole-grain crackers, and fruits will provide it. Some mothers have developed their own favorite recipes for high-energy blender drinks using ingredients such as milk, yogurt, eggs, nuts, and bananas or other fruits.

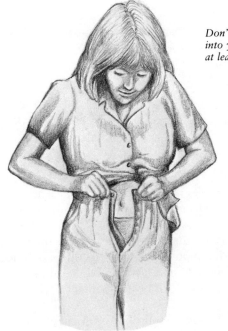

*Don't expect to be able to get into your jeans for several weeks, at least.*

Avoid snacking on foods or drinks that are high in sugar. Refined sugar provides only "empty" calories—empty, that is, of vitamins and minerals. Soda, cookies, and candy will not provide sustaining energy and may diminish your desire for more nutritious foods.

Mothers who are vegetarians can certainly maintain a diet to support their nutritional needs. But since vitamin $B_{12}$ is found only in the animal kingdom, deficiencies may occur when a mother maintains a "vegan" diet, excluding eggs and milk products as well as meat. Supplementation with up to 4 milligrams of vitamin $B_{12}$ per day is recommended.

Although nutritionists recommend that a nursing mother drink five glasses of milk a day, there is no need to drink milk if you don't like it or can't tolerate it. Although milk is an excellent source of calcium and protein, other foods can be substituted to meet these needs. Meeting the daily requirement of 1,600 milligrams of calcium may be important in preventing osteoporosis (weakened bones) later in life. Twenty-five percent of all women in the United States develop this disabling condition. Foods high in calcium are listed in the table below.

| Serving | Milligrams calcium |
|---|---|
| yogurt (8 oz.) | 288 |
| cheeses (1 oz. cheddar or swiss) | 213 |
| cottage cheese (½ cup) | 106 |
| ice cream (½ cup) | 110 |
| tofu (½ lb.) | 290 |
| salmon (3 oz.) | 207 |
| sardines (3 oz.) | 272 |
| mackerel (3 oz.) | 321 |
| broccoli (½ cup) | 68 |

Although dark green vegetables in general are rich in calcium (100 milligrams per half cup), the calcium they provide is poorly absorbed by the body. Broccoli is the one exception to this rule. If you do not drink milk or eat other dairy products, calcium supplements may be necessary. The least expensive supplement, with the highest concentration of calcium, is calcium carbonate. Avoid bone meal and dolomite, as some types have been found to be contaminated with lead.

**Dietary supplements.** If you took vitamin and iron supplements in pregnancy, it is generally recommended that you continue to take them for at least the first few months of nursing. Some nursing mothers develop vitamin B deficiencies, experiencing depression, irritability, impaired concentration, loss of appetite, and tingling or burning feet. A daily B-complex supplement is often prescribed to reverse these symptoms. Sometimes nursing mothers are advised to take brewer's yeast, a natural source of all B vitamins, iron, and protein. Some mothers feel it has improved their milk supply or has increased their overall energy level. Health-food stores carry brewer's yeast in a powdered form that can be mixed with juice or milk.

Vitamin supplements are no substitute for nutritious food, of course, and in large quantities they can sometimes be dangerous. There have been reports of fussiness in babies whose mothers take brewer's yeast or large doses of vitamin C. Vitamin $B_6$ supplements in large doses have been reported to reduce milk production.

**Foods and substances you may be wondering about.** There are no foods that should be routinely avoided by nursing mothers, but occasionally a baby will be bothered by something the mother has eaten. Some babies fuss for up to 24 hours after their mothers have eaten garlic, onions, cabbage, broccoli, brussels sprouts, cauliflower, or beans. A heavy intake of fruits, especially during the summer months, has been known to cause indigestion and diarrhea. If your baby has unusual and persistent symptoms such as sudden refusal to nurse, vomiting, diarrhea or green stools, fussiness at the breast, or colic symptoms, see the Survival Guide for the First Two Months.

Caffeine taken by the mother has been known to cause irritability and colic symptoms in some babies. Caffeine is present in coffee, tea, and many soft drinks. You may want to limit your intake of these beverages. Chocolate has also been known to bother some babies.

An occasional glass of wine or beer is not believed to harm a nursing infant. Because alcohol passes through the breast milk, however, moderation is essential.

Mothers who smoke have lower levels of vitamin C in their milk than nonsmokers. If you smoke, try to limit the amount and don't do it around the baby. Breathing cigarette fumes increases a baby's risk of contracting bronchitis and pneumonia, and perhaps of succumbing to crib death.

# Nursing Your Baby

## *Your Nursing Style*

During the early weeks, each mother develops her own style of nursing. Many women feel comfortable putting their babies to breast whenever they signal the desire to nurse. Others expect their babies to fall into a predictable feeding schedule. They may be troubled when their babies nurse irregularly or want to nurse again soon after being fed. These mothers may worry that perhaps they have too little milk or that it is somehow inadequate. Sometimes they feel they must hold the baby off until a certain number of hours have passed since the last feeding. But the breasts do not need to rest for any period of time to build up a supply for the next feeding; they produce milk constantly. The expectation that a baby should nurse on some type of a schedule usually leads to frustration for both mother and baby—and not uncommonly to breastfeeding failure.

The typical newborn infant nurses between eight and fifteen times in a 24-hour period, or about every one to three hours. Because of the ease with which breast milk is digested, nursing infants have been described as continuous feeders. Not only must a baby nurse often to satisfy his hunger and stimulate an adequate milk supply, but he also seeks out the breast to satisfy his needs for sucking, security, and comforting.

It is a common misconception that the breast empties in a certain number of minutes, and that a baby should be taken from the breast after those minutes have elapsed. In fact, many mothers experience the release of milk several times during a feeding. The average infant in the first two months nurses between 10 and 20 minutes per breast for a total feeding time of 20 to 40 minutes. The "all-business" nurser who swallows continuously with few pauses may be done in less time, whereas the "dawdler" may take up to an hour. The length of nursing time may vary in the same baby from feeding to feeding. Before long, most mothers can tell when their babies have had enough.

Some babies nurse from only one breast at a feeding some or most of the time. This is fine so long as the baby seems satisfied and is gaining weight adequately.

I strongly recommend that your baby be weighed at two weeks of age. Although many infants are not scheduled for a routine well-baby exam until three to four weeks of age, a weight check at two weeks can be very beneficial. If the baby is back to his birth weight or beyond, you can be reassured early on that your nursing relationship is progressing well. On the contrary, if the baby has not yet regained his birth weight, you can usually correct this quite easily. When a poor weight gain is not discovered until three or four weeks, it is more likely to upset everyone and may be harder to correct than it would have been at two weeks.

You may find that nursing is the most enjoyable part of your day—a time to sit back, relax, and simply enjoy being with your baby. But it may be difficult at times for you to break away from what you are doing or sit still long enough for the baby to have a leisurely nursing. It may help to make a special little nursing area for yourself—or two or three nooks in different parts of the house. You might want to include a book, some magazines, or a note pad within reach. Having the phone nearby may also be handy. Some mothers make a point of getting a snack or something to drink just before sitting down to nurse.

Many babies seem to get hungry whenever food is served. If you usually find yourself nursing while trying to eat dinner, you may find a baby swing handy. Some parents have found that taking the baby for a walk just before dinner lulls him to sleep so that they can eat without interruption.

## Your Milk Supply

During these early weeks your milk production may seem somewhat erratic. At times your breasts may feel as if they are bursting with milk. At other times you may worry there is not enough milk, especially if your breasts seem empty and your baby wants to nurse all the time. Many mothers notice this happening around two to three weeks and then again at six weeks, when a baby normally experiences appetite spurts and nurses more often to stimulate increased milk production. You can expect fluctuations in your milk supply as production becomes regulated according to the baby's demands.

By six to eight weeks postpartum, many mothers notice that their breasts seem smaller or feel less full. This does not usually mean that less milk is being produced, but only that the breasts are adjusting to the large amount of milk within and the baby's feeding pattern.

Some mothers misinterpret their babies' increased demands and their own softer breasts, and begin offering supplemental bottles. For most mothers and babies, this marks the beginning of the end of breastfeeding. The mother begins to assume that she cannot make enough milk for her baby, and she offers more and more formula instead of allowing the baby to increase her own supply of milk. After receiving formula the baby sleeps longer and nurses less often. She becomes increasingly frustrated at the breast as her mother's milk supply dwindles. For these mothers and babies, breastfeeding is soon over.

Some mothers try to satisfy their babies' hunger with solid foods. Introducing solids during these early weeks is also inappropriate. Young infants are both physiologically and developmentally unable to manage them. Their digestive systems and kidneys are not mature enough to handle cereals and other baby foods. Infants may develop allergies to solid foods given during this period because their immune systems are still immature.

Fluctuations in the fullness of your breasts and in your milk supply will probably pass by the end of the second month. In the meantime you can be reassured your milk supply is probably fine so long as you are nursing at least eight times in each 24-hour period and allowing the baby to nurse as long as she needs. For additional concerns about your milk supply see the Survival Guide for the First Two Months.

## Infant Dietary Supplements

**Vitamins.** It is generally agreed that vitamin supplements are unnecessary for the healthy, full-term infant who is breastfed. Although it was previously thought that breast milk contained little vitamin D, a water-soluble variant that appears in milk was recently discovered. Vitamin D is important for the formation of teeth and bones, and a deficiency can cause rickets. This disease, though, is rarely seen in breastfed babies. Babies who may be at risk include those with low birth weights, those with dark skin, those who are rarely exposed to the sun, and those whose mothers do not eat meat, fish, or dairy products. The recommended dose of vitamin D for these infants is 400 units per day. Twice this daily dose can be toxic.

**Iron.** The full-term newborn has sufficient stores of iron for the first four to six months after birth. The small amounts of iron in breast milk are very well utilized by the nursing infant, so iron supplementation is unnecessary. Furthermore, iron supplements can interfere with the protective properties of breast milk. The premature infant, however, is likely to use up his iron stores earlier than the full-term infant. Supplemental iron is recommended for the premature infant beginning at two months of age.

**Fluoride.** Fluoride given from early infancy is believed to reduce cavities 50 to 65 percent during childhood. Even though a mother may drink fluoridated water, little fluoride reaches the baby through the breast milk. The American Academy of Pediatrics therefore recommends that all infants receive fluoride supplements of 0.25 milligram per day.

Some authorities, however, believe fluoride supplementation is unnecessary for the breastfed infant, and point out that too much fluoride can cause spotting of the tooth enamel. Additionally, some infants are reported to become fussy and irritable and to have gastrointestinal upsets after being given fluoride.

If you prefer, you can delay fluoride supplements until your baby is four to six months of age. Fluoride is available by prescription either alone or in combination with vitamins A, C, and D (which most breastfed infants do not require).

## Illnesses: Yours and the Baby's

With minor illnesses such as colds and flu, breastfeeding need not be interrupted. Most likely your baby will have already been exposed to the virus that causes you to get sick. In fact, the antibodies you produce against the illness will reach the baby through the milk and may protect him from getting the same sickness. Even though you may not feel much like eating, try to drink extra fluids to keep from getting dehydrated. Should you need to take a medication, even an over-the-counter drug, be sure to check on its safety for the baby. Your milk supply may seem low during or just after an illness, but a few days of concentrated nursing will usually reverse a low milk supply.

Should your baby become ill, nursing should certainly continue. Breast milk is the best source of fluids and nourishment for recovery and nursing the best source of comfort. But sickness often changes a baby's nursing pattern. He may nurse more than usual, or he may lose interest in feeding.

Ear infections, sore throats, and fever blisters may make nursing painful for the baby. As long as he is nursing infrequently or is refusing to nurse, be sure to express your milk every couple of hours to keep up your supply. Colds and stuffy noses may make nursing difficult for him. Holding him upright while feeding, using a humidifier in the room, or administering nose drops prescribed by your doctor may make nursing more comfortable.

Fever is a sign of infection. During the first four months, a temperature above 99°F., if taken in the armpit, or 101°F., if taken rectally, should be reported to the baby's doctor. If, besides having an elevated temperature, the baby doesn't act like his usual self or he nurses poorly, he should be checked by your doctor. The severity of a fever does not always correspond with the seriousness of an illness; a high fever may appear with a minor infection and a low fever may accompany a serious infection. Because a fever may lead to dehydration, frequent nursing is very important.

Diarrhea in the breastfed baby, although less common and usually less severe than in the formula-fed baby, is characterized by frequent (12 or more per day), extremely loose or watery bowel movements. Often the stools are foul-smelling, and they may contain mucus or blood. Since babies lose a great deal of fluid with diarrhea, they can easily become dehydrated, making frequent nursing important. With its high water content, breast milk helps replace the lost fluids. Diarrhea generally improves within three to five days. Fever, infrequent feedings, or signs of dehydration (dry mouth, few wet diapers, listlessness) are signs to notify your doctor. In cases of severe diarrhea, doctors occasionally recommend supplements of an electrolyte solution, such as Pedialyte, in conjunction with nursing.

## The First Two Months: What's Normal?

During the first two months you can expect your baby will nurse between 8 and 15 times a day, including at least once at night. If your baby sleeps four to six hours at a stretch at night or takes a three- to four-hour nap during the day, she will probably want to nurse often during the next few hours to make up for the meal she missed. The baby who is nursing less than eight times in a 24-hour period or who is sleeping longer than six hours at a stretch at night is typically the infant who fails to gain enough weight during the early weeks of nursing.

Generally, eight or more wet diapers a day are a sign the baby is getting enough milk. By two weeks, most nursing infants have regained their birth weight. A gain of five to seven ounces a week thereafter is normal.

The breastfed baby typically has loose, watery, or seedy stools. During the first month most infants have at least one bowel movement daily. After the first month it is not uncommon for a baby to go several days without a bowel movement. As long as the baby seems comfortable there is generally no need for concern; your baby is probably not constipated or underfed. The baby who is not getting enough to eat typically has small, and usually infrequent, brown or greenish stools.

Many mothers continue to experience dripping or spraying milk during or between nursings. But some women stop leaking altogether after the first several weeks, and most gradually notice less leakage.

At some point during the first two months you will probably start to experience the sensations of milk let-down. You may notice this tingling, pins-and-needles feeling in your breasts just before or during a feeding or at any time your baby signals you with his cry.

Occasionally babies spit up after a feeding. Some babies spit up after every nursing. This is usually due to an immature digestive system; what comes up is normally just a few teaspoons. Spitting up passes with time; until it does, keep a diaper or small towel handy.

A baby cries for any of a number of reasons. She may be hungry or tired, or she may just want to suck and be held. Sucking at the breast is soothing and comforting for her. Babies usually have a fussy period in the evening. Although many theories have been suggested to explain why this is, most babies are comforted by extra nursing. Try not to assume your milk is somehow lacking. Many mothers who interpret their babies' cries this way begin supplementing with formula and soon find the babies weaned. See the Survival Guide for the First Two Months for more on why babies cry and how to cope with it.

During the appetite spurts at about two to three weeks and six weeks of age, your baby may act more fussy than usual and want to nurse more often. After a few days of frequent nursing, your milk supply will increase to meet her needs and she will return to her usual nursing pattern.

Some babies cry hard, as if they were in pain, for prolonged periods every day. They are said to have *colic,* which is just a name for extreme irritability that continues day after day—for any of a number of reasons. Some cry at the breast or refuse nursing entirely. If your baby has colic symptoms, see the Survival Guide for the First Two Months.

You may have heard that tending to your baby each time she cries will spoil her or will reinforce her behavior and cause her to cry more often. Nothing could be further from the truth. Babies do not cry to exercise their lungs, but because they are in need of something. If your baby's needs are met in infancy she will develop a sense of security, and she will grow to trust in you and others as well.

During these early weeks, while you are learning about your baby, caring for his needs, and learning to breastfeed, you are apt to experience some feelings of concern, confusion, and perhaps even inadequacy regarding your mothering abilities. Motherhood and breastfeeding may not be exactly what you expected. Your baby's crying and the unpredictability of his sleeping and wakeful periods may be upsetting. The baby's nursing schedule (or lack thereof) and his many needs may make it impossible to feel organized or productive. Some mothers may be disappointed by the lack of help from their health care providers. Early motherhood may also bring feelings of loneliness and isolation.

It is normal to have mixed feelings about nursing. Try to keep in mind that new motherhood requires a period of uncertainty and adjustment and that nursing, and mothering, gets easier with time.

# SURVIVAL GUIDE
# for the First Two Months

## Concerns about Yourself

Sore Nipples

Breast Pain

Plugged Ducts

Breast Infection (Mastitis)

Breast Abscess

Breast Lumps

Leaking Milk

Overabundant Milk

Lopsided Breasts

Depression

## Concerns about the Baby

Spitting Up and Vomiting

Pulling Away from the Breast

Refusal to Nurse

Fussiness and Colic

Getting Enough Milk

Underfeeding

# Concerns about Yourself

## Sore Nipples

It can certainly be discouraging when sore nipples persist beyond the first week. If this happens to you, review the information in the Survival Guide for the First Week. It may be helpful to have your partner, friend, or lactation professional observe your latch-on technique and compare it with the descriptions of latch-on in Chapter 2. Don't discount the possibility that your nipples are irritated due to thrush or a nipple cream, as these are frequent causes of sore nipples.

If you have suddenly developed sore nipples after a period of comfortable nursing, the most likely cause is thrush. See the Survival Guide for the First Week.

## Breast Pain

For a variety of reasons, your breasts may begin to hurt during nursing or become perpetually tender or sore. If this happens, it is important to identify the cause so that any necessary action can be taken.

Engorgement can occur any time the breasts become overly full—when the baby misses a feeding, for example, or when he begins to sleep longer at night.

Mothers usually begin noticing normal let-down sensations during these early weeks. They may be experienced as a mild ache at the start of nursing or a tingling, pins-and-needles sensation.

A deep pain, often described as "shooting," that occurs just after nursing is thought to be related to the sudden refilling of the breast. These pains disappear after the first few weeks of nursing.

Pain during nursing, often described as burning or stinging, is usually associated with thrush. The nipples may be pinker than usual. Sometimes a rash may be visible. See Thrush Nipples, Survival Guide for the First Week, for additional information on causes and treatment.

## Plugged Ducts

If you can feel a tender area or painful lump in your breast, the cause is probably a plugged milk duct. The skin over the area may be reddened. As some mothers describe it, a large part of the breast feels overly full and does not soften with nursing.

Plugged ducts are most common during the early weeks of nursing. They occur for a variety of reasons. Often a plugged duct follows a missed feeding or a long stretch at night without nursing. Too tight bras, especially underwire types, may obstruct the milk flow and lead to plugged ducts. Baby carriers with tight straps can also cause this to happen. Occasionally dried secretions on the tip of the nipple or a plug in one of the nipple openings blocks the milk flow and causes a backup of milk behind the nipple.

For unknown reasons, plugged ducts seem to be more common during the winter months. Mothers with high milk production, including mothers nursing twins, seem to be more prone to plugged ducts. Some breastfeeding specialists feel that mothers who drink an insufficient amount of fluids or who are overly fatigued may also be more susceptible to developing plugged ducts.

Plugged milk ducts do not require antibiotic treatment, but they must be taken care of promptly to prevent a breast infection from developing.

**Treatment measures for plugged ducts**

1. Remove your bra if there is any question that it may be too tight or may be pressing into part of your breast.
2. Nurse frequently, at least every two hours. Begin each nursing on the affected breast.
3. Increase your fluid intake so that you urinate more frequently.
4. Apply moist heat to the breast for 15 to 20 minutes before nursing.
5. Gently massage the breast just above the sore area while nursing. A vibrating massager works well.
6. If you are following the preceding recommendations but notice no change in your breast after a feeding or two, try positioning the baby with his chin close to the plugged duct to promote better drainage.
7. When the blockage seems to be in the nipple, look for dried milk secretions or a clogged nipple pore, which may resemble a whitehead. If necessary, you can gently remove a visible plug from a nipple opening with a sterile needle.
8. Be alert for signs of a developing breast infection—fever, chills, and achiness—so you can treat it promptly.

## Breast Infection (Mastitis)

It has been reported that up to 30 percent of all nursing women develop mastitis, or infection of the breast. It occurs most commonly in the first three months postpartum.

Mastitis causes flu-like symptoms, including fever, chills, achiness, headache, and sometimes nausea and vomiting. Normally only one breast is affected; it usually becomes swollen, tender, and reddened in a limited area.

A breast infection may follow a cracked nipple or a plugged milk duct. Other possible causes are a tight bra, skipped feedings, infrequent changing of wet breast pads, anemia, stress, and fatigue. Although doctors usually prescribe antibiotics for mastitis, many women recover quickly without them. In one study of women with mastitis, half used no antibiotic, and none of them suffered complications (Riordan and Nichols, 1990). However, an antibiotic may be necessary if your symptoms do not resolve after you've followed the treatment measures specified here, or if you are severely anemic. Otherwise you may prefer to avoid antibiotics, as they can lead to yeast infections in both mother and baby.

With prompt and proper treatment the symptoms usually subside within 24 hours. It is most important to continue nursing frequently during this period; discontinuing nursing would slow healing and might lead to the development of a breast abscess. You don't need to worry that the baby will get ill, since the infection involves only the breast tissue, not the milk. Try to identify the probable cause of the infection so you can prevent a recurrence in the future.

Mastitis in both breasts, though rare, is sometimes a sign of B-streptococcal infection, which is transmitted by the infant to the breasts. When both breasts are affected the baby's doctor should be promptly notified so that any necessary treatment of the infant can begin.

**Treatment measures for mastitis**

1. Go to bed, if you haven't already.

2. Remove your bra if you are more comfortable without it or if there is any question that it may be too tight or pressing into part of your breast.

3. Nurse frequently, at least every two hours, and begin each nursing on the affected breast. Advice to wean or temporarily discontinue nursing is based on disproven theories. Giving up nursing may slow healing and lead to a breast abscess.

4. Increase your fluid intake so you notice an increase in urination.

5. Apply moist heat to the breast for 15 to 20 minutes before nursing and intermittently between feedings.

6. Check your temperature every four hours. Acetaminophen tablets (such as Tylenol) may help reduce your fever and discomfort.

7. Some mothers report that taking 1,000 milligrams of vitamin C four times a day speeds healing and recovery.

8. If after 24 to 48 hours you feel no better, call your doctor, who will probably prescribe antibiotics. Antibiotics should be taken for the entire time they are prescribed, even though the symptoms may disappear.

9. After you have completed a course of antibiotics, watch for symptoms of yeast growth—thrush, diaper rash, or sore nipples (see the Survival Guide for the First Week).

10. See Survival Guide for Months Two through Six if you have a recurrence.

## Breast Abscess

On very rare occasions, a breast infection may develop into an abscess. A breast abscess is an accumulation of pus walled off within the breast. It may occur when a mother stops nursing during a breast infection, when treatment for mastitis is delayed, or when a mother has trouble fighting off a breast infection because she is severely anemic.

A breast abscess should be suspected whenever mastitis symptoms are prolonged beyond a couple of days and a lump persists. The lump may be hard or soft but does not change with nursing. An abscess must usually be drained by a physician, either in an office or a hospital. After it is drained, recovery is rapid.

The development and treatment of an abscess is usually a rather traumatic experience. You may be advised to stop nursing entirely, or you may doubt yourself whether you should continue. Although you need not abandon nursing completely, it may be suggested that you not nurse on the affected breast for the first few days after it is drained. In the meantime, you can use an electric pump to maintain your milk flow until the baby resumes nursing on both sides. The incision may leak milk for a short while, but it will heal and close over. I developed an abscess at six weeks postpartum and went on to nurse successfully without any further difficulties.

## Breast Lumps

Lumps in the breast are very common during the early weeks and are usually related to lactation.

The breast may feel generally lumpy when it is overly full or engorged. A sudden tender lump is usually a sign of a plugged milk duct or, when accompanied with fever and flu-like symptoms, a breast infection. A lump that appears just before nursing and seems to get smaller or disappear afterward is probably a small cyst that fills with milk.

Whenever a lump shows no change in size for longer than a week, it should be examined by a doctor. It is probably a harmless cyst or benign tumor; cancer is rarely the cause. But if your baby persistently refuses to nurse on the breast with the lump, you may have a tumor; see your doctor for a thorough breast exam as soon as possible. If further diagnosis or treatment is recommended, you don't need to wean your baby, although a doctor unfamiliar with the lactating breast may recommend weaning. Many women have undergone mammography, ultrasound, breast biopsy, and lump removal without any interruption of nursing. Feel free to get a second opinion whenever drastic measures are recommended.

## Leaking Milk

See the Survival Guide for the First Week for basic information on leaking, dripping, and spraying milk.

After a few weeks of nursing you may notice that leaking diminishes or stops entirely. This need not be a cause for concern so long as the baby is continuing to nurse frequently and is gaining weight.

But, if continuing leakage is becoming bothersome, you might want to try to stop it by pressing your wrist or the heel of your hand against your nipples whenever they start to drip. Some lactation professionals warn, however, that this practice may lead to plugged ducts during the early weeks.

If leaking at night continues to be troublesome, you might try nursing the baby just before you go to sleep.

## Overabundant Milk

Some mothers seem to produce too much milk. Aside from the jokes about being able to nurse twins, you may feel uncomfortably engorged much of the time. Leaking and spraying may be bothersome. Your baby may gasp and choke as the milk lets down.

Most women find this is less of a problem after the first two months of nursing. In the meantime, it is best not to interfere with production by taking steps to decrease your supply. Measures such as decreasing your fluid intake are not recommended. Wearing plastic breast shells or pumping after nursings usually promotes a further increase in milk supply.

If your baby has difficulty nursing because the milk lets down forcefully, see Pulling Away from the Breast. Refer to the Survival Guide for Months Two through Six if you continue to produce milk in overabundance after two months.

## Lopsided Breasts

When one breast receives more stimulation than the other, milk production in that breast increases, commonly resulting in a lopsided appearance.

Providing more stimulation to the smaller breast will usually even out the size difference between the two. Start each feeding on the smaller side for a day or so. If your baby nurses there only a few minutes, encourage her to take the smaller breast again after she has nursed at the fuller one. As soon as your breasts become closer in size, you can begin alternating the breast at which the baby begins each feeding.

## *Depression*

Most women go through emotional changes after giving birth. Some experience moodiness, anxiety, or an occasional "blue" day; a few become truly depressed. New mothers who complain they are depressed are often told their feelings are normal and to be expected. This is not true.

Some women who feel depressed after giving birth may simply be overtired or poorly fed, or they may have unrealistic expectations about themselves and their new roles. Some are overextended; others may be suffering from sudden isolation from caring adults. Depression is more common among women who have moved their households either just before or just after giving birth.

Postpartum depression (PPD) is thought to be a biochemically induced reaction in response to giving birth. Symptoms usually include several of the following:

- Change in eating habits (poor appetite or overeating);
- Change in sleep patterns (difficulty falling or staying asleep, oversleeping);
- Feeling tense, nervous, or anxious;
- Fatigue or lack of energy;
- Trouble concentrating, forgetfulness, or confusion;
- Periods of daily crying;
- Feelings of hopelessness;
- Withdrawal, lack of interest in usual activities;
- Excessive worry or guilt;
- Failure to keep postpartum check-up appointment;
- Inability to care for oneself or the baby; and
- Thoughts of death, suicide, or harm to the baby.

Some of these symptoms are common among new mothers and may be helped by the following suggestions. If you experience many of these symptoms or they become severe, you should seek professional help.

**Coping measures for depression**

1. See if your partner can take more time off work—to spend with you and the baby, or to relieve you of some of your mothering duties for a little while.
2. Evaluate your daily activities and plan for at least one nap every day. Enlist the help of your partner or friends to ensure you get the rest you need. If necessary, call an agency or find a local student to help with housework or caring for any older children.
3. Eat a well-balanced diet. A good breakfast is a must. If you have little appetite, fix small nutritious snacks for yourself throughout the day. Avoid sweets and caffeine.
4. Take time with your appearance every day. When you get up, make a point of getting dressed, fixing your hair, and putting on a little makeup, if you like it. Pamper yourself with a facial, a new hair style, or something new to wear. Looking good helps you to feel better about yourself.
5. Get some light exercise every day. Join an exercise or dance class; many offer free infant care. Take a brisk walk every day with the baby.
6. Make an effort to spend time with other adults. Invite friends over, join a postpartum group, or make friends with other mothers from your childbirth class. Your childbirth instructor may have additional suggestions. If you have just moved to the area, ask your pediatrician's or family practitioner's nurse for other resources.
7. Seek professional counseling if your symptoms are not resolving. Low-cost counseling is available in most communities at various mental health agencies. If medication is recommended, be sure it is safe for your nursing baby.

# Concerns about the Baby

## Spitting Up and Vomiting

Spitting up small amounts of breast milk is common; some babies do this after almost every nursing. Occasionally a baby may vomit what seems like an entire feeding. Although there may be no apparent cause, this can sometimes be traced to something the mother recently ate. Vomiting can also be a sign of infection. You will want to notify your doctor if the baby has a fever or if the vomiting continues.

When a baby continues vomiting forcefully after most feedings, you should suspect that either he is sensitive to something in your diet (see Something in Your Diet) or he has pyloric stenosis. *Pyloric stenosis* is an obstruction of the stomach that typically develops at about two to four weeks of age. Although this condition is most common in first-born males, it can occur in females. Typically the vomiting becomes progressively worse; the baby eventually stops gaining weight, or loses, and may become dehydrated. In the breastfed infant the condition may go undiagnosed longer than in the bottle-fed infant, since breast milk is digested much more easily than formula. The baby's weight may not be affected until the obstruction becomes nearly complete. Frequently waves can be seen moving across the baby's lower abdomen from the left side to the right just after a feeding and prior to vomiting. X-rays confirm the diagnosis. The obstruction is corrected with a relatively simple surgical procedure.

Breastfeeding can resume within a few hours after the obstruction is removed. At this time breast milk is especially good for the baby because of its digestibility. Some mothers notice a temporary reduction in the milk supply after the baby's surgery. Rest, frequent nursing, and switching the baby from side to side during the feeding usually reverse this situation.

## Pulling Away from the Breast

Babies pull off the breast while nursing for a variety of reasons. Often it is because they have had enough to eat or they need to be burped. If your baby has a cold, he may pull away because he is having trouble breathing through his nose. Try to position him so his head is elevated more during nursing. A cool-mist vaporizer may help to thin the nasal secretions so he will breathe easier.

Some babies pull away from the breast gasping and choking as the milk suddenly lets down. This is usually a temporary problem; the baby gradually learns to keep up with the rapid flow of milk. In the meantime, positioning the baby differently may help. Try sitting the baby up, using the football hold, or lying on your back with the baby's head over you. Some mothers manually express or pump milk until the initial spray has subsided. If your baby pulls away from the breast and cries or refuses to nurse, see Refusal to Nurse, as follows.

## Refusal to Nurse

If your baby pulls away from the breast crying or refuses to nurse, don't assume she is ready to wean. There are a number of possible reasons for such behavior, but when it persists, it can frequently be traced to certain foods in the mother's diet that are causing an allergic response in the baby. Typically this starts around two weeks of age. The baby usually acts fussy and colicky; she may have greenish stools, or she may spit up or vomit. Other symptoms may include gassiness, redness around the rectum, a mild rash anywhere on the body, or a stuffy nose. Fussiness while nursing and refusal to nurse may increase as the day goes on. Although the baby refuses the breast, she may eagerly take breast milk from a bottle. The reason for this is unclear.

A baby who has developed a yeast infection (thrush) may also become fussy at the breast and refuse to nurse. Besides the characteristic white coating in the baby's mouth, you may notice she is gassy and somewhat cranky. You may also notice a bright red, dotted or peeling rash on her bottom or on your nipples. Your nipples may burn or itch.

Occasionally a baby will refuse to nurse if the mother's milk has developed a strong and unpleasant taste due to a particularly spicy food she has recently eaten. Deodorant and perfume sprays have also been identified as causing some babies to refuse the breast.

Finally, a baby may refuse to nurse any time she is not feeling well. Ear infections and other discomforts commonly cause this behavior.

### Treatment measures when the baby refuses to nurse

1. As long as your baby refuses to nurse, manually express or pump your milk every two to three hours so your supply will not be affected. Feed the baby by bottle.
2. Taste your milk a few times to determine if a food you may have recently eaten has flavored the milk. If you notice a strong peppery aftertaste, try to identify a spicy food you may have eaten. In the meantime, pump until the baby resumes nursing (usually 12 hours or less).
3. Check your baby's mouth and your nipples for signs of thrush. See the Survival Guide for the First Week. Treatment with gentian violet is not effective for this problem.
4. If you think your baby may be having an allergic response, see Something in Your Diet.
5. If your baby is irritable and refuses to nurse, and you can find no reason for it, have the baby examined by your doctor. An ear infection or other discomfort may be causing your baby to act this way.

## Fussiness and Colic

You may be surprised to learn how much crying a baby can do and how uncomfortable it can make you feel. The sound of a baby's cry is intended to be distressing, so adults will be alerted to his needs and answer them.

All babies have fussy periods during their early weeks. You will probably notice that your baby is more fussy at around two to three weeks and again at around six weeks, when most babies experience appetite spurts. Fussiness in the late afternoon or evening is typical.

Many mothers tend to blame themselves for their babies' crying, wondering if their inexperience, nervous feelings, or milk supply is somehow responsible. Keep in mind that most babies fuss and seek out the comfort of the breast when they are tired, bored, lonely, or uncomfortable as well as when they are hungry. For unknown reasons, some babies simply need to suck more than others. Even if your baby is nursing double time, try not to think your milk supply is inadequate. When babies are having appetite spurts, they increase their nursing frequency for a few days to stimulate increased milk production. See Getting Enough Milk if your are worried the baby is not getting enough to eat.

**Coping measures for fussiness**

1. Offer your breast—it is a source of comfort as well as nourishment for your baby.

2. Pacifiers are soothing to many babies who need lots of extra sucking, who are fussy, or who have difficulty calming themselves. If your baby doesn't take a pacifier at first, try different kinds. Offer the baby one every few days.

3. Be sure to burp your baby frequently while he nurses or sucks on a pacifier.

4. Some babies are comforted by being swaddled tightly in a light blanket.

5. Warm baths with the baby may be soothing to both of you.

6. Most babies love motion. Try walking, using a front baby pack or stroller. Rocking can also be comforting—borrow a rocking chair if you don't already have one. You can put a small baby in a baby swing if you bolster him with towels or blankets. Most babies are lulled to sleep by car rides.

7. Noise may calm a crying baby. A radio in the baby's room, a tape recording of a humming car, vacuum cleaner, or vibrator, or an aquarium near the baby's bed may help him sleep.

8. Consider sleeping with the baby if you aren't already.

9. Take a short break from the baby each day. Your partner might play with the baby while you take a bath, go for a walk, or visit a friend.

10. Find another mother who has a fussy baby. There's nothing like a friend who really understands.

**More serious crying.** Some babies are extremely irritable and fussy during the early weeks. They have periods of intense crying, when it seems something must be terribly wrong. Such babies are said to have colic—but this is only a catch-all term for an unidentifiable discomfort.

If your baby's crying makes you feel that something is wrong, trust your instincts. By all means have your baby examined by your doctor. Outlined below are common reasons I have identified for periods of intense crying in infants. I highly recommend the book *Crying Baby, Sleepless Nights* by Sandy Jones (see Suggested Supplemental Reading) as an excellent resource for parents of fussy babies.

*Swallowing excessive air.* Some babies swallow a great deal of air when nursing or sucking on a pacifier. When this air passes through the intestines the baby can be quite uncomfortable. If your baby is passing a lot of gas, make an effort to burp her more frequently. Try to get a burp at the start of each feeding as well as several times during it. If you give the baby a pacifier, she will need extra burping. Do not allow the baby to suck on a bottle nipple in place of a pacifier, even if the open end is taped or stuffed with cotton.

*Diaper rash.* A baby may fuss a lot if she has a diaper rash. For an entire day, apply a zinc oxide ointment (such as Desitin); expose the baby's bottom to the air as much as possible, and leave off disposable diapers or plastic pants. The rash should improve dramatically, unless it is caused by yeast. A yeast diaper rash is a dotty, red rash or a peeling rash that resembles a mild burn.

*Yeast infection.* Although they are common in infants, yeast infections are frequently overlooked as the cause of excessive fussiness. A baby with a yeast infection usually shows signs in his mouth—on his tongue, inner lips or cheeks, or gums. This is known as thrush. The baby is typically very gassy, as the yeast is frequently present in the intestinal tract as well. The yeast may also cause a diaper rash, as just described. The mother's nipples are often reddened; they may show a rash, and they may itch or burn. One nipple may be more affected than the other.

Nystatin suspension (Mycostatin) is the drug of choice if your baby has a yeast infection. Because the nystatin is swallowed, the yeast in the bowel will be eliminated. Treatment with gentian violet kills only yeast in the mouth and therefore is not recommended for the baby who is fussy and gassy unless the nystatin seems ineffective after several days of treatment. See Thrush Nipples, Survival Guide for the First Week, for a complete discussion of treatment measures.

Mycostatin Ointment can be used to treat the baby's diaper rash; it can also be used on your nipples. If your baby has no rash it would not be unusual for one to appear shortly after treatment with the oral medication. If the baby does have a rash, don't be surprised if it gets worse during the first few days of treatment.

If the baby's stools are green, he may also be reacting to certain foods in his mother's diet. See Something in Your Diet, as follows.

*Something in your diet.* Caffeine is well known to cause irritability in some infants. Coffees, teas, and many soft drinks contain caffeine. Chocolate contains a caffeine-like substance that can also cause a reaction in a baby. Additionally, many headache and cold remedies include caffeine or another bothersome chemical, phenylpropanolamine.

Other commonly consumed substances have also been implicated in causing problems for some infants. Artificial sweeteners are one example. Disturbances in the baby's intestinal tract may be caused by laxatives taken by the mother. Certain dietary supplements taken by the mother or given directly to the baby, such as brewer's yeast, fluoride, and large doses of vitamin C, have been known to cause diarrhea and allergic reactions.

Occasionally a mother notices that a certain food she eats upsets her baby. Foods most commonly reported to make babies fussy include fruit and fruit juices in large amounts, some types of fish, peanuts and peanut butter, and gas-producing vegetables such as beans, cabbage, and onions.

If your baby is fussy day after day, she may actually be allergic to certain foods you are eating. A baby who is having an allergic reaction to foods typically has greenish stools or more than six yellow stools a day. The stools may also be bloody or foul smelling. Other common symptoms of food allergy include gassiness and redness around the anus. Some of these babies have mild rashes, on the face, neck, or shoulders; some have stuffy noses. They may frequently spit up or occasionally vomit.

Some allergic babies, their mothers report, fuss while nursing or sometimes refuse to nurse. But these babies will usually take pumped or manually expressed breast milk from a bottle. They often nurse best during the night.

Eliminating only one food at a time from your diet is not likely to give you a true picture of what's bothering your baby—it may be more than one food. If you suspect your baby is allergic to something you are eating, eliminate the most common allergenic foods for one week. This means cutting out all dairy products (such as milk, cheese, butter, yogurt, ice cream), citrus (oranges, lemons), tomatoes, pineapples, eggs, and peanuts from your diet. (Wheat and corn are also possible, but less common, offenders.) If you eat a lot of fruit or drink a lot of juice, cut back. Be sure to read all labels carefully since eggs and milk are hidden in many prepared foods.

If your baby is allergic to some or all of these foods, you should notice dramatic improvement before the week is out. After a week or so, see how the baby reacts when you eat one of the suspected foods.

Try peanut butter or citrus fruit first. If the baby isn't bothered, feel free to add that food to your diet again. After another week try eggs. Continue trying one food each week until you have identified just which foods bother your baby. Some mothers have found that even small amounts of the offending foods cause severe symptoms in their babies, whereas other mothers have discovered they can have a little milk, ice cream, or cheese every four or five days without the baby being too bothered. (If you must cut out dairy products from your diet, be sure you are taking sufficient calcium in another form; see Chapter 4).

If your baby does not get better on your elimination diet, you might try cutting out wheat and corn as well. If that doesn't work, you could contact an allergist for allergy testing. Also consider whether your baby might be troubled with hyperlactation syndrome.

*Hyperlactation syndrome.* Recently researchers have identified a kind of colic that is characterized by gassiness, frequent stools, spitting up, and general discomfort and fussiness (Woolridge and Fisher, 1988). While these babies may seem to be allergic to something in their mother's diet, they show little or no improvement with the elimination of common allergens. Typically these babies nurse frequently from both breasts and are gaining weight above the expected norm. Their mothers often have an overabundant milk supply.

The underlying cause of the colic is thought to be the baby's disproportionate intake of the low-fat foremilk, the milk that is available early in the feeding. When a baby consumes large amounts of foremilk and little of the fatty hindmilk, his stomach rapidly empties, dumping excess lactose into the bowel. This results in increased fermentation and colic symptoms.

Relief of the colic is achieved by getting the baby to empty the breast at each feeding so that he receives not only the foremilk but the fatty hindmilk too. The baby should be allowed to nurse from the first breast until he spontaneously pulls away satisfied. He should not be interrupted at any point to be switched over to the second breast. Some authorities feel that until the colic subsides the baby should in fact be offered just one breast per feeding and should be limited to that side for one and a half to two hours before nursing on the other side.

*The baby's temperament.* Every baby is born with his own distinct personality. Some babies tend to be quiet, whereas others are more active. Some babies are highly sensitive to their surroundings, overreacting to any sudden stimulation. They are tense and jumpy, and often fussy. They may go almost instantly from sleep to calm to full-blown crying. Once crying, they may be difficult to soothe. Although some of these babies need to be carried around or entertained continually, others may actually resist being held or cuddled.

Learning how to mother a highly sensitive baby takes time and patience. You will soon develop a sense of what your baby enjoys and what he does not, how much stimulation he can tolerate and how to help him settle down. If your baby does not enjoy touching, try not to take it personally. With time and a gradual increase in physical closeness, he will eventually be able to tolerate and enjoy being held. Most babies outgrow their early fussy months and go on to be happy children.

## Getting Enough Milk

For any number of reasons, you may be wondering if your baby is getting enough to eat. It may be that she seems to be nursing all the time or is especially fussy. Frequently mothers worry about their milk supply in the evening, especially when their babies are around two to three weeks and six weeks old. At these times babies experience appetite spurts and demand to be fed more often; frequent nursing is normal and necessary to stimulate increased milk production.

You can't tell whether your baby is getting enough breast milk by offering her a supplemental bottle of water or formula after nursing. Most babies will take a few ounces from a bottle even when they are full. Your baby is most likely getting enough milk if—

- She is nursing at least eight times in a 24-hour period.
- You can hear her swallow while she is nursing.
- Your breasts seem to be softer after nursing.
- The baby is wetting eight or more diapers in a 24-hour period.
- The baby has bowel movements daily during the first month, or passes large yellow stools every few days after the first month.

If you need further reassurance, have your baby weighed. The nurse in your doctor's office will probably be happy to do this for you. By two weeks of age, your baby should have regained her birth weight. Thereafter, an adequate weight gain is anywhere between five and seven ounces a week.

Signs that your baby may not be getting enough to eat include all or most of the following:

- The baby is nursing less than eight times in a 24-hour period.
- She is sleeping six hours or longer at night without nursing.
- She swallows infrequently while nursing.

- She is excessively fussy or apathetic and sleepy most of the time.
- She is wetting fewer than seven diapers in a 24-hour period.
- She is passing small and infrequent stools.

If your baby shows all or most of these signs, notify your doctor for a weight check and read the following section, Underfeeding.

## Underfeeding

It is upsetting and even frightening to discover that your new baby is not gaining weight normally. You may wonder about your ability to produce milk—but this is usually not the problem.

Most babies who fail to gain weight are nursing too infrequently or too briefly. The breastfed baby should nurse at least eight times in a 24-hour period, including at least one feeding at night during the early weeks. The average baby nurses 10 to 20 minutes at each breast, or about 20 to 40 minutes at a feeding. Infants who pause frequently or for long periods during a feeding may take even longer to complete. Some babies are "lazy sucklers"—they sleep six straight hours or longer at night, suck inefficiently at the breast, and usually nurse with their eyes closed. Babies with thrush sometimes develop this nursing pattern. Your baby should be thoroughly examined to make sure there is no other reason he is not gaining weight.

Most likely, your baby's problem can be remedied without your calling a stop to nursing. It will be much easier if you have the support of your doctor and your partner. If possible, see a lactation professional.

Offering your baby formula will probably put more weight on him, but unfortunately it will not correct the nursing problem. When supplementing with bottles of formula begins, nursing usually soon ends.

Let your doctor know you want to continue nursing and would like to try to correct the problem without supplementing with formula at first. Arrange for another weight check in five to seven days.

### Treatment measures for underfeeding

1. Try to find out for yourself where the problem lies. Has the baby been nursing frequently enough? Think about your baby's nursing style. Does he pause a lot and nurse too briefly to get a full meal? Might he be a "lazy suckler"? Is he sleeping for excessively long periods at night? Taking short, choppy sucks instead of long, drawing ones? Nursing with his eyes closed? Does he have thrush in his mouth?

2. If the baby uses a pacifier, put it away.

3. If you can, spend a couple of days in bed with the baby. If this is impossible, at least take things slower for several days; nap once or twice a day when the baby naps.

4. Nurse your baby frequently—every two hours during the day and evening and every three hours at night. This may mean waking the baby. Undress him down to his diaper to increase his interest and vigor.

5. Nurse for 30 to 45 minutes per feeding. Watch your baby suck and listen to him swallow. As soon as his swallowing begins to taper off, or his sucks become short and choppy, switch breasts. The first day or so you may need to switch breasts every two to three minutes. This is one of the most effective ways to improve your baby's sucking and stimulate milk production.

6. Burp your baby several times during each feeding. Some babies feel full, and therefore refuse the breast, when they have air in their stomachs.

7. Drink fluids to satisfy your thirst. Taking brewer's yeast may also be helpful. But do keep in mind that frequent, effective nursing is most important in maintaining and improving your milk supply.

8. Don't feel guilty! Chances are that if your baby had a different mother the same thing would have happened. Don't hesitate to contact a lactation professional for support and guidance.

Within 48 to 72 hours of increased stimulation, your breasts should feel fuller. The baby's weight should increase sufficiently within four to six days. But don't weigh the baby before and after feedings or even daily—the results may be distorted and disappointing. Once your baby is gaining five to seven ounces a week, you can relax your schedule somewhat, but weigh the baby weekly for a while until he is gaining steadily.

If your baby has lost a significant amount of weight or is dehydrated, or if your doctor insists on supplementation, consider one of the following methods. First, you can nurse your baby every two hours as just outlined, then pump your milk, switching back and forth for about twenty minutes. An electric pump is most effective. Use this milk to supplement nursing along with any necessary formula. If it is difficult to interest your baby in nursing as often as every two hours, limit the amount of formula to one or one and a half ounces per feeding. Once you notice your breasts are fuller, stop supplementing, and follow the course of action already described.

Second, you can use a nursing supplementation device. With this device you can nurse the baby and provide supplementation at the same time, avoiding the bottle altogether. Again, it is essential to nurse frequently, switching the baby back and forth during each feeding. Some mothers have found that by switching the baby back and forth for 30 minutes and then using the supplementation device for 10 minutes more, they have increased the milk supply and ensured the baby has gotten enough to eat. (See Appendix A for more information on nursing supplementation devices.)

**If treatment fails.** It is frightening to suddenly realize that your new baby has lost an excessive amount of weight or has not gained enough. Although the techniques just outlined will reverse the situation for most mothers and babies within several days, occasionally they won't work. This may be because the problem has gone unrecognized too long. Usually the underlying cause is the baby's faulty suck or a poor nursing pattern. The longer a baby has failed to stimulate adequate milk production the more difficult it can be to correct the problem, and the longer it can take.

A few mothers simply fail to produce milk. Women who have had certain types of breast surgery may fall into this category (see Nursing After Breast Surgery, Chapter 3). Another group of women who cannot produce milk are those with insufficient glandular tissue. These women experience no breast enlargement during pregnancy, often have one breast that is significantly smaller than the other, and experience no fullness on the third to fifth postpartum day (see Chapter 3). A lack of support from family, friends, and professionals can only make matters worse. Even with all the best information and support, things sometimes don't turn out as we hope.

If you have given it your best but finally end up having to bottle-feed, you have not failed as a mother. Be proud of your efforts to nurse, and concentrate on providing your baby with all the cuddling and loving that you can.

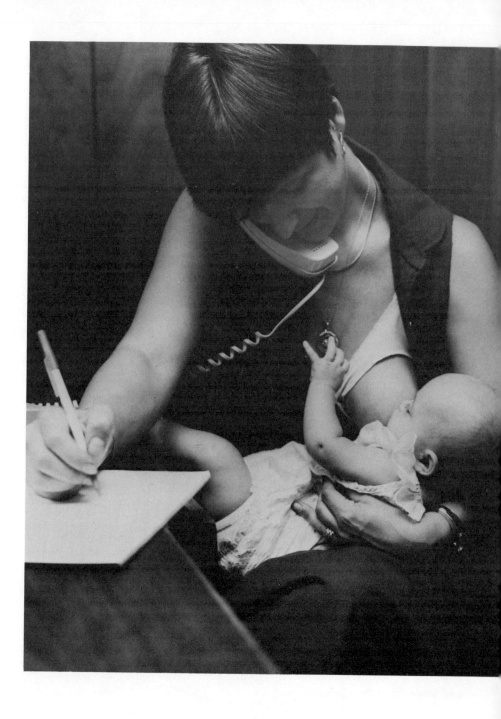

# CHAPTER FIVE

# Traveling Together, Being Apart

## Taking the Baby Along

## Occasional Separations

## Returning to Work or School

Work Options
Choosing a Caregiver
Choosing an Expression Method
Introducing a Bottle
Collecting and Storing Your Milk
Back at Work

TODAY'S NURSING MOTHER IS OUT AND ABOUT, TAKING CARE OF BUSI-ness, enjoying the company of friends, returning to work or school, taking time out for fun. In many ways, nursing simplifies life considerably. With the increasing acceptance and popularity of breast-feeding, more and more mothers are able to nurse their babies while participating in a wide variety of activities.

# Taking the Baby Along

Your nursing baby can go with you almost anywhere—and with a lot less hassle than you would face if you were fussing with formula and bottles.

You may feel comfortable nursing in the presence of family or friends you are visiting, or you may be a bit uneasy. You can always retreat to the bedroom, of course, but that's not much fun. Learning to nurse discreetly and without embarrassment will put most people at ease. You might want to practice ahead of time getting the baby on your breast with a blanket or shawl draped over your shoulder and the baby's head. If you wear a shirt or a sweater you can pull up, or if you unbutton your blouse from the bottom, you will expose less of yourself. Most maternity shops carry a line of attractive tops and dresses designed for discreet nursing.

If you are going out for the day or spending a few hours in town, you may want to nurse just before you leave. A couple of diapers and a few moist wipes in a sandwich bag, and you're off. If you are using a cloth baby carrier, you may find it easier to put it on before you go.

After a couple of hours out, look around for a comfortable place to sit with your baby. Many mothers feel comfortable nursing in public places and are hardly noticed when they do so. Some stores and restaurants have dressing rooms or pleasant restrooms where you may prefer to feed the baby.

Mothers appreciate the ease of taking long trips with their nursing babies. Most young infants travel well in a car. (Of course, the baby should always ride in a car seat approved for safety, no matter how short the trip.) You will want to stop every few hours for nursing and a diaper change. If the baby's car seat faces backward, you may be able to manage nursing while sitting in the back seat next to her.

The older baby may be less happy in the car seat for long periods. Whenever possible try to start long stretches in the car just before nap time. Try hanging some of the baby's toys on her car seat or keeping a bag of toys and other fun things in the back seat.

If you are planning to fly, you might try to reserve bulkhead seating;

this will give you extra space, though you won't be able to keep your carry-on luggage at hand. Try to choose a flight that is lightly booked. This way you are more likely to get an empty seat next to you for more room and privacy. Nursing during takeoff and landing will help the baby's ears adjust to the changing air pressure. If you must fly when the baby has a cold, give her a safe antihistamine an hour before takeoff.

# Being Apart

## Occasional Separations

Any number of situations may come up in which you must be separated from your baby—an evening out, perhaps, a family or career obligation, or a stay in the hospital.

When you plan to be away from the baby for just a few hours, you can manually express or pump some milk for him ahead of time. The best time to collect milk is just after nursing, especially if the baby has nursed from just one breast. In this way you will not lessen the amount of milk available for the baby at his next feeding. Getting an ounce or so after the baby nurses is typical. You will need to collect milk several times for each feeding you'll miss, as most babies take about three to four ounces at a bottle feeding. If you will be away longer than four to five hours, bring the pump along; you will need it to prevent engorgement and to keep up milk production (see Choosing an Expression Method and Collecting and Storing Your Milk, in this chapter).

If you will be separated from the baby for a day or longer, you may be able to store enough milk for him ahead of time. If not, you can substitute a commercially prepared formula. While you are away, try to pump at least every two and a half to three hours to maintain your milk supply. Renting an electric pump may be more convenient for you. If possible, freeze the milk you pump while you are apart so that it can be used later.

Hospitalization of a nursing mother rarely necessitates weaning, even though some doctors advise it. Some hospitals have electric breast pumps available for nursing mothers. If your hospital doesn't, you can rent a pump and take it with you, or have one brought in. You may be able to arrange for the baby to be brought in for nursing visits, or even for the baby to stay with you (providing you, a family member, or a friend can care for him). If you will be manually expressing or pumping your milk, try to do so frequently to maintain your supply. Ask the nursing staff to refrigerate your milk so that it can be taken home for your baby.

Questions may arise about the safety of medications you need to take in the hospital. Although most medications pass through the breast milk, the majority are safe for nursing babies. Occasionally a doctor may be unsure whether a given medication is safe for a baby, and so recommends weaning when the question arises. You can check the safety of the drug yourself in Appendix B. If a drug is not considered safe for a nursing baby, you can continue to pump your milk, discarding it until the medication is no longer required.

# Returning to Work or School

Not so long ago, a new mother planning to return to work might never have considered nursing her baby or would have decided to wean near the end of her maternity leave. Today, with the growing number of working women and the increasing awareness of the many benefits breastfeeding offers, more and more mothers are choosing to nurse their babies while continuing with their careers.

Your extra efforts to continue nursing are well worth it. The cost of formula aside, breastfed babies are generally healthier. The less your baby is sick, the less time you must spend away from work or school. Nursing also saves you time and energy, which is especially important when you are combining the responsibilities of employment and family. Perhaps most important, nursing helps you maintain the close, loving relationship you have with your baby. Many mothers who work outside the home or attend school feel that breastfeeding offers emotional compensation for the hours that must be spent apart. The security of your breast comforts the baby and helps make the time you are together special and rewarding for both of you.

## Work Options

Although there may be no question in your mind that you will be returning to work or school after your baby is born, you are lucky if you have some flexibility in determining the length of your maternity leave. Your time at home after giving birth is important for both you and the baby: it is the time in which you will get to know each other and form a special tie between you. It will also be a time for you to rest and recover from the physical stress of the birth process. Some women need a little while, and some need a long while, before they are ready to add the demands of work or school. Breastfeeding experts have noted that mothers who stay home for 16 weeks or longer experience fewer difficulties maintaining their milk supply once back at work.

Because you cannot know just how you will feel after you deliver, explore what options may be open to you ahead of time. Depending on your financial situation and your work demands, you may be able to arrange for an extended leave, beyond the usual six to eight weeks. Or you may be able to arrange to work at home, return to work part time, take fewer classes, or share your job with another person. Each of these options has worked well for many mothers.

Part-time work offers many advantages to the nursing mother. Fewer hours apart means fewer missed feedings, lower child care costs, and generally less hardship for both mother and baby.

Your employer also benefits by agreeing to shorter hours. Replacing an employee is time consuming and costly, especially if she has special skills that are an asset to the organization. Besides, part-time employees are known to be just as productive as those who work full time, if not more so. They tend to stay out sick less often, and they generally waste less time when they are at work. Part-timers can also help to reduce the overtime hours employers must pay for. You might agree to come in fewer hours each day, or fewer full-hour days. Both arrangements have advantages and drawbacks for the nursing mother.

Of course, part-time work also means part-time pay. Perhaps the only choice for you is full-time work. Still, a somewhat flexible arrangement may be possible. With a "flextime" schedule, you might work eight hours a day but remain free to start earlier or later than normal. This system could allow you to spend a leisurely morning with the baby and perhaps get a few chores done. You might also be able to reduce the number of hours that the baby must be left with someone else if your partner can pick her up when he gets off work.

Some mothers arrange to take their babies to work with them. Although this is not possible for most women, it can be managed in some work settings. Another option is child care at the work site. Some employers and employees have found this to be an ideal arrangement. If you work with other parents of infants or small children, it might be well worth looking into this possibility.

Another possibility is having the baby brought to you for nursings, or going to the baby yourself during your lunch hour. Usually, the major obstacle in having the baby come to your work place is finding someone willing and able to bring her. If you choose to go and spend your lunch hour with the baby, you will need to find child care close to your work place. Combining your coffee breaks with your lunch hour may give you enough time to leisurely manage travel time, nursing, and eating.

## Choosing a Caregiver

Finding just the right person to care for your baby can make all the difference in your state of mind while you are away. You may have the good fortune of relying on your partner or another loving relative to provide child care. Although this can be an ideal arrangement that makes the separation easier on both mother and baby, for most of us it is not an option.

If you will be shopping for a caregiver, be sure to start early so you can take your time. You may prefer that the caregiver come to your home, or that you take the baby to her. If you decide on taking the latter arrangement, try to locate a caregiver who lives close to your place of work or school. This will help you minimize the time you are apart and will be more convenient if you decide to nurse during your lunch breaks. You may prefer someone who will care for your baby alone, or you may be willing to share the caregiver's services with others.

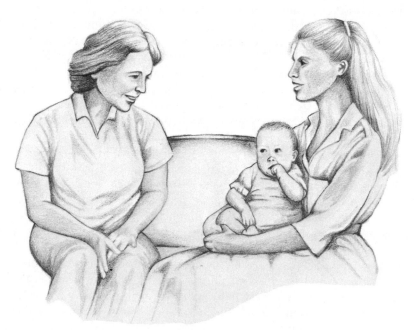

Let each prospective caregiver know about your nursing relationship and your own particular style of caring for the baby. Be sure to ask for the names and telephone numbers of other families whose children she has cared for in the past or is caring for now. It's also a good idea to try to find out if she can make a long-term commitment to your baby; having to suddenly find a replacement can be upsetting for both you and your baby. If she cares for other children, try to schedule your meeting for when they will be present. This will give you the opportunity to observe firsthand the caregiver's style, and to see whether your baby would receive enough individual love and attention in the setting. In some states, child care providers are licensed and limited in the number of infants and children they can care for. Feel free to ask about this.

In making your final choice of who will care for your baby, trust your intuition. If something doesn't feel quite right, look elsewhere. Before making a final commitment, be sure to discuss how you will handle illness (either your baby's or the caregiver's), who is to be called in an emergency, how much advance notice is necessary if the baby will be absent or late, fees and when they will be due, and any written agreements.

You may consider having the baby spend several hours or a full day with the caregiver a week or so before you go back to work or school. Such a "trial run" may be reassuring for you, or you may feel, as many mothers do, that the first separation should occur only when the situation demands it.

## Choosing an Expression Method

If you will be missing one or more feedings while you are away at work or school, you should plan to manually express or pump your milk. This will help to prevent engorgement and, more important, to maintain your milk supply. The milk can be used later to feed your baby while you are away. A mother who leaves her baby for longer than four to five hours a day and does not manually express or pump her milk, particularly if the baby is younger than six months, usually finds that the supply lessens until it no longer meets the baby's needs when mother and baby are together.

(If your baby is older than six months and is eating solid foods, you may decide against expressing your milk while you are apart. Bottle or cup feeding of formula, or of whole milk if the baby is a year or older, may be substituted while you are at work.)

*When using hand expression, catch the milk in a cup or any other clean container.*

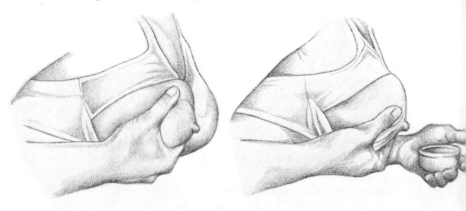

**Manual expression.** Many mothers feel that expressing milk by hand is more convenient and natural than using a pump. You can learn this technique while nursing, practicing on the free side when the baby stimulates the milk to let down. Place a towel in front of you to catch the spray as you get started. Position your thumb and index finger about one and a half inches behind the nipple, where the milk sinuses are located. Push your fingers straight back toward your chest and then squeeze them together with a slight rolling motion, lifting the nipple outward. Avoid sliding your fingers away from their original position. With several practice sessions most mothers can master manual expression. Once you have the motion down, rotate your fingers around the nipple to empty other milk sinuses.

When you begin expressing milk away from the baby, you will probably find that a few moments of gentle breast massage will stimulate the milk to let down. Catch the milk in any clean container. To get a greater amount, switch back and forth from one side to the other as soon as you notice the flow lessening. You can save time by expressing milk from both breasts at once, into containers on a table in front of you. Once you have learned how, the whole process should take about twenty minutes.

In recent years breast pumps have become increasingly popular with nursing mothers. There are three basic types of pumps: hand-operated, battery-operated, and plug-in. Since each pump has its own unique features, you will need to find the one that is best suited to your particular needs.

**Hand-operated pumps.** These are portable and relatively inexpensive; the best are also comfortable and easy to use. They are ideal for mothers who need a pump only occasionally. Listed as follows are the major hand pumps on the market.

*bicycle horn pump*

*"Bicycle horn" pumps.* These are widely available for under ten dollars in most drugstores. A bulb is squeezed for suction, and the milk flows directly into it. Most authorities warn against using milk collected this way, since the bulb is difficult to clean and may harbor harmful bacteria. Many women find, moreover, that these pumps do not work well and can be uncomfortable. When used improperly, they can cause trauma to the breast or the nipple. And since they hold little milk, they must be emptied frequently.

*Evenflo Breast Pump*

*Evenflo Breast Pump.* A variation of the bicycle horn pump, the Evenflo pump is available for under ten dollars in most drugstores. Many mothers complain that this pump is inefficient and uncomfortable. Also, the bulb may become contaminated with bacteria.

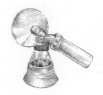

*Evenflo Natural Mother Pump.* Available for about $22 in many drugstores, this pump creates suction by use of a plunger that is pulled outward.

*Evenflo Natural Mother Pump*

*Nurture Pump.* The Nurture Pump has a soft silicone breast funnel that massages the areola when suction is created with the bulb. The manufacturers boast that their pump mimics the sucking action of a baby better than others and draws milk with a higher fat content. Although not available in stores, the Nurture Pump is available from Lact-Assist, Inc., 4026 Woodmont Boulevard, Nashville, Tennessee 37205 for $40 plus $1.25 for shipping. Call 615-371-8984.

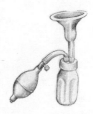

*Nurture Pump*

*Ora'lac Pump.* Designed by a nursing mother, this pump can be used more discreetly than others. The mother sucks on a tube to create the suction and release. Some mothers have found the device a bit tipsy. The Ora'lac Pump is available through some drugstores and from the company. Send $30 (includes shipping and tax) to Ora'lac Pump, Inc., Box 2400, Sitka, Alaska 99835. Phone 907-747-8270.

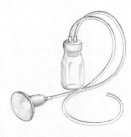

*Ora'lac Pump*

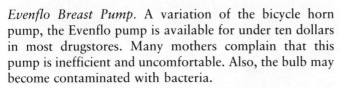

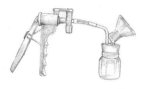

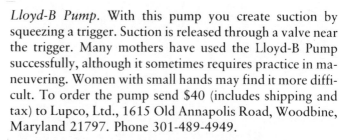

*Lloyd-B Pump*

*Lloyd-B Pump.* With this pump you create suction by squeezing a trigger. Suction is released through a valve near the trigger. Many mothers have used the Lloyd-B Pump successfully, although it sometimes requires practice in maneuvering. Women with small hands may find it more difficult. To order the pump send $40 (includes shipping and tax) to Lupco, Ltd., 1615 Old Annapolis Road, Woodbine, Maryland 21797. Phone 301-489-4949.

*Cylinder pumps.* Available in many drug and discount stores as well as maternity shops, cylinder pumps are very popular with nursing mothers. They consist of two plastic cylinders. Suction is created by sliding the outer cylinder away from the breast, starting with short, frequent pulls to initiate the milk flow. If the head of the pump is not angled, the mother may need to lean slightly forward. After two or three ounces are collected, it is usually necessary to empty the milk into another container. Cylinder pumps range in price from about fifteen to twenty-five dollars. There are many brands on the market, but the following are tried and true.

*angled-head cylinder pump*

- *Egnell Hand Breast Pump.* This angled-head pump is available from Egnell, Inc., Cary, Illinois 60013. Call toll free 800-323-8750; Illinois, Alaska, and Hawaii residents call collect 312-639-2900.
- *Comfort Plus (Marshall-Kaneson) Breast Pump.* This straight-head pump is available in many drugstores, discount stores, and baby stores. For replacement parts, write or call Marshall Electronics, Inc., Lincolnshire, Illinois 60069. Phone toll free 800-323-1482 (in Illinois, call 312-634-6300).

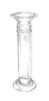

*straight-head cylinder pump*

*Medela Manualectric Breast Pump.* This pump creates a gentle suction when the plunger is pulled outward; the release is automatic. The milk flows into the attached bottle. The pump can be easily adapted for use as a milk receptacle with an electric pump. A minor disadvantage is that the pump cannot be stood up for storage. The Medela pump is available from Medela pump rental stations and from Medela, Inc., P.O. Box 386, Crystal Lake, Illinois 60014 for about twenty-five dollars. Phone toll free 800-435-8316; from Illinois, Alaska, or Hawaii phone collect 815-455-6920.

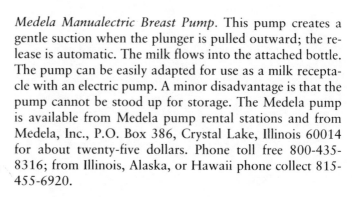

*Medela Manualectric Pump*

**Battery-operated pumps.** Relatively new on the market, these are more expensive than hand-operated pumps, and they require only one hand to use. Many mothers report, though, that the batteries need to be replaced rather often, and at this writing the pumps seem to have a high rate of breakdown. Four battery-operated pumps are currently available.

*Gentle Expressions Pump.* Made in Japan, this pump uses two AA batteries to produce a constant suction, which can be regulated. The suction is released by pressing a small button on the side of the pump. Because the suction builds slowly, some mothers have found the pump rather ineffective. The Gentle Expressions Pump can be ordered from Healthteam, 627 Montrose Avenue, South Plainfield, New Jersey 07080 for $39.95 plus $3.50 shipping. Phone orders are accepted; call 201-561-4100.

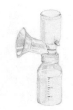

*Gentle Expressions Pump*

*Egnell Lact-B Pump.* This Swiss-made pump uses two AA batteries to produce suction, which is released by pressing a bar on the front of the pump. One slight disadvantage is that it is difficult to see the milk flow into the pump. This pump is available from Egnell, Inc., Cary, Illinois 60013, and from many of Egnell's breast pump rental stations. Call toll free 800-323-8750; Illinois, Alaska, and Hawaii residents call collect 312-639-2900.

*Egnell Lact-B Pump*

*Mag-Mag Pump.* This battery-operated pump is available with an optional AC adaptor. You can find it for about $47 ($59 with AC adaptor) at drugstores, discount stores, and many baby stores. Accessory parts are available from Marshall Electronics, Inc., Lincolnshire, Illinois 60069. Phone toll free 800-323-1482 (in Illinois, 312-634-6300).

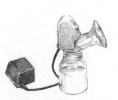

*Mag-Mag Pump*

*Evenflo Natural Mother Sof-Touch Ultra Pump.* Available in drugstores, this battery-operated pump uses longer lasting C batteries and has an optional AC adaptor. This pump also offers a flexible silicon breast funnel. The suction on this pump seems to build and release rather slowly. The cost is about $40.

*Evenflo Natural Mother Sof-Touch Ultra Pump*

**Plug-in pumps.** The final type of breast pump runs on electricity from a wall socket. These pumps have several advantages over hand-held pumps. In addition to requiring less effort generally, they require only one hand to operate.

This means you can pump while reading, talking on the phone, or eating lunch. Most mothers find the pumps gentle yet very efficient, and some feel they work somewhat faster than hand-operated pumps.

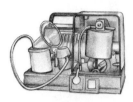

*automatic pump*

Fully automatic pumps create a regular suck-release pattern that closely approximates the sucking action of a baby, and they promote very efficient letdown. Most fully automatic pumps now offer optional double-pump kits so that both breasts can be pumped at the same time. Double pumping can significantly cut the amount of time needed to empty both breasts; also, studies have suggested that more milk is obtained using the double-pump kit. A fully automatic pump is preferable if you are pumping frequently for a baby who is not nursing or if you are working full time. Such a pump is less portable than other kinds, however, and is also more expensive to buy. But you can rent one instead (and long-term rental rates are about a third the cost of formula feeding).

Semiautomatic pumps also run on electricity from a wall socket, but the mother uses her finger to create the suction. These pumps are available for purchase only. Although they are less expensive to buy than fully automatic pumps, they may be less efficient, and therefore less suitable for the mother who is pumping full time.

*Egnell Electric Pump.* Although this automatic pump costs around a thousand dollars to buy, it is widely available through rental stations for about $2.25 per day. A long-term rental rate of one dollar per day is available when the pump is used for four months or more. Double-pump kits are also available. Contact Egnell, Inc., Cary, Illinois 60013 to locate a rental station near you. Call toll free 800-323-8750; from Illinois, Alaska, or Hawaii call collect 312-639-2900.

*Medela Electric (015) Pump.* This automatic pump is also widely available through rental stations for about $2.25 per day. The company offers a reduced rate of 99 cents per day if you rent the pump for at least five months and pay in advance (a three-month rate is also available). Like Egnell, Medela also offers an optional double-pump kit. Contact Medela, Inc., P.O. Box 386, Crystal Lake, Illinois 60014. Call toll free 800-435-8316; from Illinois, Alaska, or Hawaii call collect 815-455-6920.

*Kadan KM-1 Pump.* This semiautomatic pump is small and portable. About the size of an electric can opener, it comes with a carrying case. Suction is generated by simply placing a finger over the vacuum release hole located on the breast shield. The pump costs about $210, as of this writing. To locate the dealer closest to you call D. A. Kadan, Inc., toll free at 800-DA-KADAN.

*Medela Lactina Electric (016E) Pump.* Medela has managed to produce a fully automatic pump that weighs just four pounds, ideal for mothers returning to work. The Lactina 016R is a six-pound version with an optional battery pack for mothers without an electricity source. Both pumps are available for rent with long-term rates and double-pump kits. The pump may also be purchased for about four hundred dollars. Contact Medela, Inc., P.O. Box 386, Crystal Lake, Illinois 60014. Call toll free 800-435-8316; from Illinois, Alaska, or Hawaii call collect 815-455-6920.

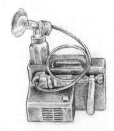

*Medela Lactina Electric (016E) Pump*

*White River Electric Pump.* White River's electric pump comes with a soft silicon breast funnel and can be used as fully automatic or as semiautomatic with finger control. It is available through pump rental stations; call 800-824-6351.

*Precious Care Pump.* This semiautomatic electric pump, new from Gerber, is about the size of a small aquarium pump. Again, suction is generated by placing a finger over the vacuum release hole. Two disadvantages are the unusually shaped breast funnel and the low suction strength. At this writing, the pump can be found in some drugstores for about fifty dollars or ordered from the Sears catalog for $44.99.

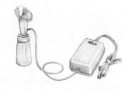

*Precious Care Pump*

*Nurture III Pump.* Also semiautomatic and the size of an aquarium pump, Nurture III has several worthwhile features: variable suction strength, optional double-pumping capability, and a one-year warranty. The Nurture III can be ordered for $85 plus $2 shipping (add $10 for a double-pump kit) from Bailey Medical Engineering, 1820 Donna, Los Osos, California 93402. Phone orders are accepted; call 805-528-5781.

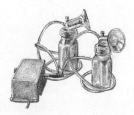

*Nurture III Pump*

## Introducing a Bottle

Getting your baby used to a bottle is important if she will be fed by someone else while you are away at work or school. It is best to wait until she is three to four weeks old before introducing a bottle. By this time nursing should be well established, so the bottle will not interfere with the baby's interest in the breast. Some babies refuse the bottle if it is first offered much after they are one month old.

It is generally best if someone other than the mother bottle-feeds the baby. You can manually express or pump your milk instead of nursing, then have your partner or someone else feed the milk to the baby. Most infants will continue to accept a bottle if it is offered about once or twice a week. Offering a bottle periodically will also give you the opportunity to practice manual expression or become proficient with your pump.

If you have waited longer than a month and the baby refuses to take a bottle, be sure to have someone else try. Frequently a baby is more confused and upset by the bottle when her mother tries to persuade her. Trying to force the baby is upsetting for everyone, and rarely successful. Some parents have succeeded by offering the bottle while walking with the baby. Hold the baby facing away from you and bounce her gently as you walk. Some babies dislike the taste of formula; try breast milk instead. Tasteless silicon nipples may be more readily accepted than rubber types.

The baby who refuses a bottle may do surprisingly well with an ordinary cup. Some parents have had success using a nursing supplementation device (see Appendix A). The soft tube is taped to the end of the feeder's finger, typically the index finger. The finger, nail side down, is then offered to the baby to suck on.

## Collecting and Storing Your Milk

Most mothers who will be manually expressing or pumping their milk while away feel more secure if they collect and store a backup supply of milk ahead of time. You can safely store it in the freezer compartment of your refrigerator for up to three months. If you have access to a deep freezer you can store it there for six months or longer.

If you plan to store your milk in the freezer compartment, collect it in clean plastic containers; small plastic baby bottles or the disposable plastic liners used with some bottles work well. Hard plastic or glass bottles are preferable for storing milk in a deep freezer. Because the entire amount must be used once breast milk is thawed, you will want to store small amounts in each container to prevent waste. If you are not sure how much milk your baby will want at each feeding, put about three ounces in each bag or bottle. Leave some room at the top of the container to allow for the expansion that occurs with freezing. Secure bottle liners by twisting the tops, bending them over, and closing the ends with rubber bands or twist ties. Be sure to label each container with the date collected.

If you wish to add more milk to some that is already frozen, chill it first in the refrigerator for about half an hour to keep the top layer of frozen milk from defrosting.

Frozen breast milk may take on a yellow color. This does not mean that is has gone bad.

The best time to collect milk for storage depends on your baby's routine. You may need to pump after a few feedings each day if he nurses frequently around the clock; you may get only an ounce or two each time. But if your baby sleeps for five or six hours at night you may be able to collect a few ounces of milk just before you go to bed or early in the morning, depending on what time he begins his sleep stretch.

While you are collecting milk at home you are also becoming more proficient at hand expression or pumping. Occasionally a mother finds that the pump she has purchased does not work well for her. If this happens, be sure to review the manufacturer's instructions and check to see that all the parts are present and properly connected. Most pumps require some practice, but if you are not happy with yours, try a different style.

When expressing your milk either by hand or with a pump, switch from one breast to the other as soon as the flow starts to diminish. This is the most effective way to stimulate more milk flow. Massaging the breasts just before and during expression encourages milk let-down and also increases milk flow.

A small proportion of women have trouble getting their milk to let down while they are pumping. A more efficient pump usually improves the situation; a fully automatic electric pump with double-pumping capability is best. If you still have difficulty even with one of these pumps, an oxytocin nasal spray (Syntocinon) will be beneficial. This is the same hormone that is naturally secreted during breastfeeding to cause the milk to release. A spray or two into the nostril a minute before pumping will provoke the let-down. Syntocinon is available by prescription only. Ask your doctor to prescribe the 5-milliliter size, which costs about thirty dollars.

At work or school, you will need a time and a place to collect your milk. Almost any private place will do—an empty office, an unused room, or the women's lounge. Talk to your supervisor if you need to

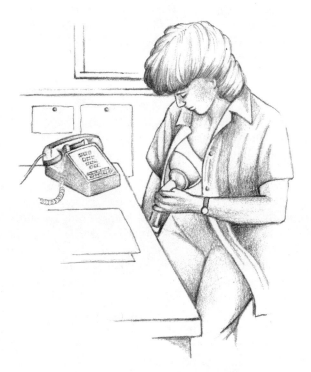

make special arrangements for regular or extended breaks. You may need to deduct the time from your usual hours or make it up at the end of the day.

You will also need a place to store your milk. Investigate whether a refrigerator is available. If there is no refrigerator, you can take a small cooler with refreezable plastic ice packs inside. Milk stays cold for several hours in these coolers, which are also handy for transporting milk home or to the caregiver's. Coolers specially made for storing and transporting breast milk are commercially available (see Appendix A).

When you pick up the baby at the caregiver's house, you can leave milk in the refrigerator for the next day. Fresh refrigerated milk is best for the baby, since it retains more antibodies than frozen milk. If the milk will not be used the following day, however, it should be labeled with the date and frozen.

You will want to thoroughly instruct whoever is caring for the baby on how the milk is to be stored and prepared. Specific written guidelines, like those that follow, are most helpful.

**Refrigerated Milk**

Use refrigerated milk within 48 hours. Take the milk out from the refrigerator just before using. Gradually, over 5 to 10 minutes, warm the milk to room temperature in a container of warm water. Do not warm the milk in a microwave or on the stove.

**Frozen Milk**

Use milk within three months if it has been stored in the freezer compartment of a refrigerator. Milk stored in a deep freezer is good for six months or longer. Always use the oldest milk first. Thaw the milk either in the refrigerator, where it can remain up to 24 hours, or in water just before feeding, gradually increasing the temperature from cool to warm. Do not defrost the milk in a microwave or over the stove. Whatever milk the baby does not take must be discarded. Breast milk cannot be refrozen.

The caregiver should be encouraged to schedule the baby's feedings so that he will be ready to nurse as soon as you arrive. This generally means the baby should last be fed about two to three hours before you are expected.

## Back at Work

Once you are back at work, you will discover what routines work best for you, the baby, and your milk supply. Nursing twice in the morning before you leave the baby is ideal. Some mothers find that bringing the baby to bed with them, if she isn't already there, and nursing an hour or so before getting up works well. You can nurse again just before you leave home or when you get to the caregiver's house. While you are at work, try to express milk about as often as you would be nursing at home. This means at least two expression sessions if you will be gone a full eight hours—three is even better.

After work, you may want to nurse at the caregiver's house before going home. Many mothers find this provides a welcome opportunity to relax and talk with the caregiver about the baby's day.

When you are at home, of course, you will want to nurse as much as possible. Some mothers encourage their baby to nurse more frequently during the evening and night; they find this helps to keep their milk supply plentiful.

Some mothers find they are unable to express as much milk as the baby needs while they are away. In this situation there are several measures to take. You can try to express milk more frequently while you are at work. This might be easier if you rent an electric pump for a while. You should be sure to switch from one breast to the other frequently as you express if you are pumping with a single collector. Using an electric pump with a double-pump kit may help you to obtain greater milk volumes. While you are nursing, you should switch the baby from one breast to the other whenever you hear his swallows becoming farther apart. You might want to consider spending a weekend in bed with the baby nursing frequently. Some mothers also stimulate increased milk production by pumping for a few minutes after nursing.

Even if you follow all the other measures, if you cannot express milk more often at work you may find that the baby needs a supplement when you are away. This may be formula, but if the baby is four to six months old and seems ready for solids, you may want the caregiver to begin introducing them.

Some mothers leak milk while they are at work. You may need to wear thick pads in your bra; keep an extra supply of them with you. Wearing printed blouses or keeping an extra jacket or sweater at work will help hide any wetness. Some mothers prefer to use plastic breast shells to keep their clothes dry. Although this usually serves the purpose, keep in mind that these cups can encourage further leaking. The milk they catch should not be saved for the baby.

If you and your partner are both working, you may be too overwhelmed by chores to cuddle and enjoy the baby as much as you would like during your hours at home. Perhaps you can afford to pay someone to come every week or so to catch up on the housecleaning.

Combining nursing and working takes a great deal of time and energy. Aside from the responsibilities of your job, the baby, and the rest of your family, it is very important that you take time to care for yourself. Nursing mothers need to eat well. Although it may be tempting to skip breakfast or lunch, most women who do this find they have little energy to meet the many demands of the day. Get up a little earlier, if you must, to fix a nutritious breakfast. Bring snacks such as yogurt, cheese, nuts, and fruit to eat throughout the work day. Some mothers find brewer's yeast gives them an energy boost and helps keep up the milk supply. To avoid constipation and plugged milk ducts, you will also need to drink plenty of fluids while you are at work. Finally, rest is essential. Most working and nursing mothers find they must go to bed earlier every night than they once did. If you can, take an hour's nap just before dinner, and nap on your days at home with the baby.

# CHAPTER SIX

# *The Reward Period: From Two to Six Months*

Caring for Yourself
Making Love
Nursing Your Baby
Starting Solid Foods

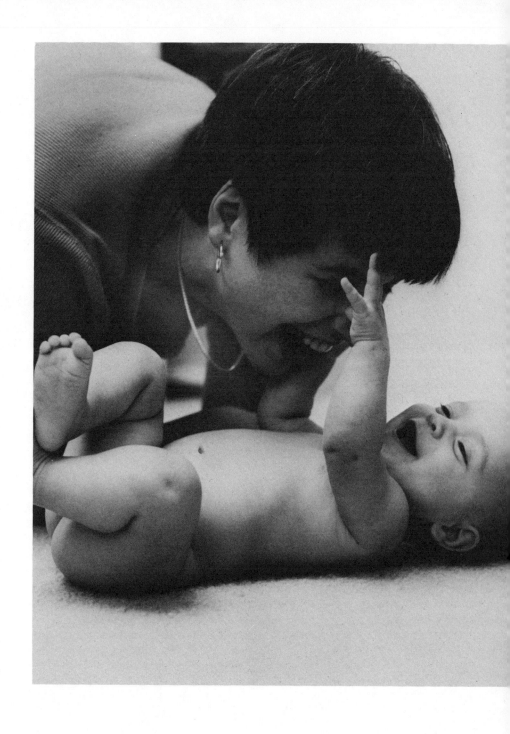

THE PERIOD BETWEEN THE BABY'S SECOND AND SIXTH MONTHS IS EX-
citing and rewarding. With the newborn stage behind, most mothers
feel relaxed and confident. The baby is more predictable, his needs
easier to interpret. By three months, his crying lessens considerably.
Day by day, the baby becomes more sociable and attuned to the people and things around him. Still, nursings are an important part of his
day, intervals for nurture and nourishment at the breast.

## Caring for Yourself

During this time, I hope, you are beginning to feel more like your
usual self. Napping whenever possible is still important, especially if
your baby is waking at night for feedings or if your energy seems low.
Your intake of food and drink continues to be essential to your overall
well-being. Neglecting your need for fluids could lead to constipation
and, possibly, recurrent plugged milk ducts. Skipping meals or substituting "empty" calorie foods for more nutritious ones could result in
fatigue and rapid weight loss. If you are overweight, limit your weight
loss to one pound per week; crash dieting could decrease your milk
supply. Most nursing mothers lose weight gradually without worrying
about snacks or calories, whereas others find that eating three regular,
satisfying meals and limiting high-calorie snacks and beverages, such
as juices and soft drinks, helps them to achieve their weekly goal.

## Making Love

After the birth of a baby most couples need time to readjust to each
other sexually. You can probably resume intercourse by the sixth-
week postpartum exam. In the meantime, you and your partner can
enjoy physical loving such as cuddling, kissing, massage, and fondling.
If your perineum feels fine and you want to have intercourse at three
or four weeks postpartum, there is no reason to wait. But you may
not yet feel ready even when your doctor, nurse, or midwife gives you
the go-ahead.

　　You may be worried that intercourse will be painful. If you have
had an episiotomy, you may feel some initial tenderness and tightness,
but your stitches should be completely healed after one month. Relaxing as much as possible will help make lovemaking more comfortable
the first few times. A warm bath, a glass of wine, and extra time with
foreplay may be helpful. Be sure to use a generous amount of lubricat-
ing gel, such as K-Y Lubricant or a contraceptive gel, in and around
your vagina. You may also want to experiment with different positions, especially if you have had an episiotomy. Some women prefer

to be on top so that they control the degree of penetration. Others find that a side-lying position feels best at first.

Most new mothers experience some vaginal dryness during lovemaking because of the hormonal changes that occur after giving birth. The vaginal secretions increase once regular ovulation resumes. Ovulation is generally delayed during nursing, for a variable period. Until your periods resume, a water-soluble lubricant can make intercourse more comfortable and pleasurable.

The breasts need not be off limits when making love. Some women, however, find them less sensitive to stimulation during the nursing period; they may also feel tender during the early weeks, and later on just after nursing. Breast stimulation and orgasm may cause the milk to let down and leak or spray. If leaking milk is bothersome for you or your partner, you might nurse shortly before you make love, or wear a blouse, a bra, or a nightgown during lovemaking.

For some time after having a baby, many women find they have less interest in making love than formerly. There are a variety of reasons for this. Estrogen, which influences a woman's sex drive as well as the amount of vaginal secretions, is produced in lower levels after she gives birth. Sometimes having so much skin-to-skin contact with the baby all day dampens a woman's desire for more physical contact. A new mother may also fear another pregnancy—whether or not the recent one was planned. At the end of the day, too, a mother may be just too tired for lovemaking.

New fathers also suffer from overwork and night wakings. Like their partners, they may be too exhausted to make love, and they may also worry about having another baby too soon.

It is important that your intimacy as a couple continues. As with most other changes in life, talking over your feelings and making some readjustments will make this period easier.

Finding the time to make love can be difficult, especially when you are tired. You may need to plan times to be together when you are rested and when the baby is likely to be asleep. Making love early in the morning or when the baby is napping may work the best. Perhaps you can take a nap in the afternoon so you will have more energy for your partner in the evening. Having the baby sleep in another room may help you to feel more comfortable.

But if neither you nor your partner is much inclined to have frequent intercourse, don't feel there is something wrong with you—your physical and emotional intimacy can continue without it. Passionate feelings will probably come easier as the baby gets older. Remember, you have a lifetime ahead of you to share your love.

**Contraception.** If you are concerned about the possibility of getting pregnant, talk over birth control options with your partner and your health care provider. Although breastfeeding delays the onset of ovulation and menstruation, and tends to postpone pregnancy, you should not depend upon it to prevent pregnancy. Whether nursing mothers should take the pill is controversial. Full-dose and even low-dose birth control pills often decrease milk production. Some doctors recommend the progestin-only pill (the mini-pill) for nursing mothers because it has little effect on milk production, yet other authorities are against the use of any pill during the nursing period because of possible long-term effects on the baby. Foam, sponges, condoms, IUDs, diaphragms, and cervical caps are all considered safe during nursing. (If you used a diaphragm or cervical cap prior to your pregnancy, it will need to be refitted now.) Some women prefer to track their natural cycles, abstaining from intercourse around the time of ovulation, but this method may be unreliable during lactation. If you prefer to use the "rhythm method," try to get personal instruction in it. Learn to keep track of all three basic body measures: basal body temperature, cervical mucus, and length of menstrual cycle.

## Nursing Your Baby

As your baby quickly grows and develops you will notice her nursing pattern also changes. You can expect two more appetite spurts during this period, the first at about two and a half to three months and the second between four and a half and six months. As with the earlier appetite spurts, the baby will nurse more frequently for a few days to stimulate an increase in milk production. Most mothers produce 30 to 36 ounces of milk or more each day during this period, a 50 to 80 percent increase over the first month.

By three or four months of age, many babies have dropped a feeding or two and are nursing about seven or eight times a day. Less frequent nursing results in decreased milk production and slowed weight gain for the baby. This most commonly occurs when a baby spends much of her day sucking on her fingers or on a pacifier. It can also happen when a working mother does not express milk frequently enough while she is away. Some babies prefer to nurse from just one breast at each feeding. So long as the baby seems content and is continuing to gain weight (close to an ounce per day) this is normal.

You may also notice that your baby is nursing for shorter periods. She can now get a large quantity of milk quickly because both she and your breasts have become so efficient. At four to five months, a baby also becomes easily distracted during nursing. At any new, sudden, or interesting sight or sound, she pulls away from the breast to look around. This does not mean she has lost interest in nursing. After several weeks she will no longer have to interrupt herself to check out what's going on around her; she'll turn her head with the nipple still in her mouth. In the meantime, you may find that nursing in a quiet or semi-darkened room helps the baby to complete her feedings.

Most three- to six-month-old babies are chubby; some may be quite plump. Parents and sometimes even doctors may become concerned about the baby who gains weight above the norm. These babies usually slow their growth during the second half of the first year and typically begin to slim down during toddlerhood. It is not advisable to restrict the baby's nursing because of his weight.

About half of all infants are sleeping through the night—that is, for a six- to seven-hour stretch—by three to four months. Many infants, both breastfed and bottle-fed, continue to need night feedings until they are six months or even older. Feeding the baby formula, cereal, or other solid foods in the evening will not help her to sleep longer at night.

Sometimes babies who have been sleeping through the night begin waking again for feedings. This can occur when a baby decreases the number of nursings during the day either because she gets distracted or because she spends too much more time sucking her fingers or a pacifier. To encourage your baby to get more of her milk during the day, try offering the breast in a quiet, darkened room or whenever she begins sucking her fingers—and limit the use of a pacifier.

Sudden night waking may be due to the discomfort of teething. Other signs of teething may include general fussiness, drooling, changes in nursing pattern, biting and finger sucking. Giving the baby a cold washcloth or a chilled water-filled teething ring to bite on may make her more comfortable. Some doctors also recommend the use of gum gels and acetaminophen drops (such as Infants' Tylenol or Tempra). An ear infection may also be the reason for sudden night waking. If your baby has recently had a cold (or a previous ear infection), beware that his ears may be the problem, even if he has no fever and isn't pulling on them.

## Starting Solid Foods

Probably no area of infant development attracts as much confusion and range of opinion as the starting of solid foods. Your family, friends, and child care advisors probably all have different ideas on when and how to begin giving solid foods to your baby. By far the most sensible approach I have found is that of Ellyn Satter, a nutritionist who breastfed her own three children. I highly recommend her book *Child of Mine: Feeding with Love and Good Sense* (1986).

Solid foods are best introduced when a baby becomes developmentally ready for them and is able to benefit from the nutrition they offer. Although this does not happen until a baby is four to six months of age, many mothers feel pressured to begin solids earlier. Some think of feeding solids as a sort of status symbol, something to brag about.

Offering solids prematurely means replacing breast milk, which is nutritionally perfect, with foods that are nutritionally incomplete. Additionally, the early introduction of solids may lead to obesity (perhaps lifelong), allergic reactions, decreased milk production, and early weaning. Rest assured, your milk provides all the nutrients your baby needs for at least the first four to six months after birth. Besides, holding off on solids is practical: the closer to six months you introduce them, the more likely you will be able to skip the "baby food" stage and start with table foods.

Some mothers go to the opposite extreme: they feel they should delay solids until eight to twelve months to prevent allergies and excessive weight gain. But obesity should not be a problem if a baby is over four months and seems ready for solids. You don't need to worry about allergies, either, if you avoid foods that are commonly allergenic—such as wheat, egg white, citrus fruits, and dairy products—and any foods to which members of your family are allergic.

You'll know your baby is developmentally ready for solid foods when he can sit with support, control his head and neck movements, and tell you he is hungry or full by leaning forward with an open mouth or pulling away and turning his head. He may indicate his readiness for solids by grabbing food off your plate or out of your hand.

At this time he will also begin to lose his tongue-thrust reflex, which causes him to push anything in his mouth forward and out. This means he will be better able to eat from a spoon, move the food to the back of his mouth, and swallow. The baby's digestive system will also be mature enough to handle solids at this time. His kidneys will be able to excrete the waste products of solid foods, and he will be less likely to develop allergic reactions from them. His iron stores will lessen, so the iron from solid foods will be beneficial for him.

When your baby is close to six months old, you may begin to notice that he still seems hungry after nursing. If after a few days of stepped-up nursings he still seems unsatisfied, feel free to experiment with solids. Occasionally the weight gain of a four- to five-month-old begins to fall off. If it does not pick up after a week or so of more frequent nursings, it may be time to begin solids.

Quite a variety of foods have been recommended as the first solids for infants: fruits, vegetables, meats, yogurt, egg yolks, cottage cheese. But all of these foods contain either too much carbohydrate, protein, or fat, or too little iron.

An iron-fortified baby cereal mixed with breast milk is the ideal first food for a baby. It meets both his nutritional and his developmental needs. Cereal meets the baby's increased demand for iron that occurs around six months. Mixing the cereal with milk provides a good proportion of carbohydrate, protein, and fat. The texture of cereal can be adjusted to match the baby's ability with semisoft food.

Rice or barley cereal is less likely to cause an allergic reaction than wheat or a mixed-grain cereal, and is therefore a better first food (be sure to check the label, as some rice cereals do contain other grains). Although they are sometimes recommended for infants, cereals that must be cooked do not contain as much iron as dry baby cereals, and what iron they do contain is not nearly as well absorbed. Ready-made baby cereals in jars also have less iron than the dry versions, and are more expensive. High-protein cereals provide more protein than young infants need.

Mix dry baby cereal with breast milk, formula, or evaporated milk diluted one to one with water. You can use whole milk (less than eight ounces a day) if your baby is six months or older and you are not concerned about an allergic response. Breast milk or a hypoallergenic formula (soy-based or predigested) is probably the best choice if you are concerned about allergies. Mixing the cereal with water or juice will not provide protein and fat for the baby.

Nurse your baby before offering cereal or another solid food. It is important to do this until he is eating three regular meals of table food, some time after eight months of age. Until then, breast milk will continue to be his most important food.

Begin with one feeding of cereal a day. At first, mix one teaspoon of cereal with enough milk to make a thin paste. At the first few feedings, don't be surprised if your baby pushes back out almost as much as you have put in. It may take a little time before he learns to move the food to the back of his mouth and then swallow it. Should your baby become upset and refuse to eat, wait a few days before trying again.

Gradually increase the amount of cereal you give at each feeding, and add a second feeding so the baby is getting a total of one-half cup of mixed cereal a day. Thicken the mixture as his eating ability improves. If you are giving supplemental iron, stop when the baby is taking one-third to one-half cup of mixed cereal a day.

For advice on adding fruits, juices, and other foods to the baby's diet, see Chapter 7.

# SURVIVAL GUIDE
# for Months Two through Six

## Concerns about Yourself

Recurrent Plugged Ducts and Breast Infections
Overabundant Milk

## Concerns about the Baby

Biting
Slow Weight Gain
One-Sided Nursing
Sudden Refusal to Nurse

# Concerns about Yourself

## *Recurrent Plugged Ducts and Breast Infections*

Many nursing mothers experience recurrent plugged ducts or breast infections. If you are suffering from either at the moment, carefully review the information in the Survival Guide for the First Two Months. If you have had more than two or three episodes, the following suggestions may be helpful in preventing more.

### Treatment measures for recurrent plugged ducts and breast infections

1. Be sure you are nursing the baby frequently at both breasts. Avoid skipping or delaying feedings. Wake the baby at night if your breasts feel too full. To encourage complete drainage of the milk ducts, massage your breasts gently while nursing. Pick a quiet place to nurse if your baby gets distracted during feedings.

2. Change nursing pads whenever they become wet.

3. Consider whether vigorous upper arm movements, such as in aerobic dancing, vacuuming, raking, or scrubbing, might be bringing on your plugged ducts or mastitis; some researchers suspect this possibility. If you think such movements are the cause, don't work so hard.

4. Get as much rest as possible. Nap whenever you can. Consider sleeping with the baby if you aren't already.

5. Snack between meals on high-protein foods.

6. Make sure you are getting plenty to drink every day.

7. Check your bra and any other restrictive clothing you may be wearing.

8. Avoid pressing against your breasts to stop leaking milk.

9. If your doctor prescribes antibiotics, take the entire course. A ten-day prescription may be needed; a five- or seven-day course may be insufficient for complete treatment.

10. If an infection recurs in the same part of the breast shortly after antibiotic therapy has ended, the antibiotic may be ineffective. Some antibiotics do not penetrate breast tissue as well as others. Be sure to discuss this possibility with your doctor or pharmacist.

11. Taking a daily iron supplement is important if you are anemic.

12. Many lactation professionals believe vitamin C supplements may help prevent recurrences of breast infections. Some suggest that taking supplemental lecithin and avoiding saturated fats in the diet may prevent plugged milk ducts.

13. A high salt intake has been implicated in increasing susceptibility to infections. Some women seem to be prone to breast infections premenstrually; this may have to do with the fact that they retain water just before their periods. Try limiting your salt intake for several days before your period is due.

## *Overabundant Milk*

Some mothers continue to be bothered by an oversupply of milk after two months postpartum. You are not necessarily producing too much milk, however, if you leak or become engorged during the baby's long sleep stretches. Only if you are still feeling uncomfortably engorged most of the time should you consider taking steps to decrease your milk supply. These measures are not recommended if you are having recurrent plugged milk ducts or breast infections.

### Treatment measures for an overabundance of milk

1. Continue drinking plenty of fluids.
2. Should you be caught in a routine of expressing milk while nursing full time, gradually decrease the amount of milk you take until you are no longer expressing any.
3. If you are not expressing routinely and still have too much milk, nurse your baby at just one breast per feeding. Let him suck as long as he likes on one side. If you become uncomfortable, express a small amount of milk from the other breast. Switch breasts with each feeding.

# Concerns about the Baby

## *Biting*

Being bitten by a baby while nursing is a common yet unforgettable experience. Naturally, you let out a holler, take the baby from the breast, and tell her "No!" Just the right thing to do.

A baby most commonly bites before her teeth come in, perhaps because her gums are sore. She is likely to try it at the end of a feeding or when she is just snacking; she may have a playful look on her face as she goes about it. This behavior may continue for as long as three or four days, but it usually ends as suddenly as it began.

Some mothers fear their babies will start biting once the first teeth have come in. This occasionally happens, but it is usually because other areas of the gums are sore, and not because the baby wants to try out her new incisors. While the baby is sucking, the tongue protects you by covering the lower teeth.

### Coping measures for biting

1. Keep your finger ready to end the feeding. Watch for a change in your baby's nursing pattern; as soon as she stops taking long even sucks and begins short choppy ones, end the feeding. If you notice a playful look on her face, end the feeding.

2. Should you miss the cues and get bit, say "No!" and end the feeding. Do not pick up the baby again to nurse for at least half an hour.

3. Avoid letting the baby snack at the breast during this period of biting.

4. Offer the baby a cold wash cloth or a chilled water-filled teething ring to chew on just before feedings.

## Slow Weight Gain

A baby is considered a slow gainer when he puts on four ounces or less a week. Three to four months is a common age for some babies to fall off in their weight gain.

Typically, these babies have decreased the number of nursings to fewer than seven or eight a day. They are often nursing less because they are sucking more on their fingers or on pacifiers. Besides lengthening the time between feedings, they have usually also shortened each feeding. They may or may not be waking to nurse at night.

A baby may also lose some interest in nursing when juices or solid foods have been introduced prematurely. Slow weight gain may occur, too, when a working mother does not manually express or pump her milk often enough while she is away from the baby, leading to an overall decrease in her milk supply. When a mother is eating too little, her milk supply may drop as well. Birth control pills, even the low-dose kind, often decrease milk production.

### Treatment measures for slow weight gain

1. Devote at least two to three days to nursing the baby and doing little else. Put the pacifier aside, and each time you notice the baby beginning to suck a finger offer the breast. You may find yourself nursing every hour or so, although increasing feedings to eight or more per 24 hours is usually sufficient to quickly increase milk production. If your baby is sleeping through the night, try to include at least one late evening feeding. You might also consider waking the baby for a feeding after he has slept five or six hours.

2. While the baby is nursing, listen for swallowing. As soon as you notice the swallowing taper off, switch breasts. Continue switching back and forth for as long as the baby is willing to continue, ideally at least 10 minutes. If the baby is easily distracted, nurse in a quiet, darkened room.

3. Should your baby refuse to nurse as often as every two hours or resist switching back and forth, you might consider expressing or pumping milk after each nursing to stimulate an increase in milk production. An electric pump may be most convenient. After two or three days of this regime, both the baby's nursing pattern and your milk supply should begin to improve.

4. If you are working, try to spend two or more consecutive days at home following the recommendations just given. While you are at work, express milk as often as possible. If you cannot express milk often enough, you may

need to supplement with formula on days you are with the baby. Some mothers feel that a nursing supplementation device rather than a bottle is more convenient and less disruptive to nursing when supplementation becomes necessary (see Appendix A).

5. After two or three days of stepped-up nursing, you should notice that your breasts feel fuller and that the baby swallows over a longer period during feedings. Continue nursing frequently, at least eight times a day. Have the baby's weight checked after a week of frequent nursing, and again a week after that. If the baby gains four to five ounces a week, everyone should be reassured that things are going well. If he doesn't, supplementation with an ounce or two of formula after some of the feedings may be necessary. You can add cereal to his diet, once or twice daily *after* nursing, if the baby is four months or older.

## One-Sided Nursing

Occasionally a baby develops a preference for one breast over the other. Perhaps the favored breast produces more milk or lets it down more rapidly. Sometimes there is no apparent reason—the baby simply prefers one side. Twins usually choose opposite sides.

Sometimes a mother unknowingly nurses the baby more at one breast, increasing its milk production. Some mothers prefer nursing on one side only; in certain cultures one-sided nursing is common.

One breast can fully support a baby's nutritional needs. But if a single baby nurses substantially more at one breast than at the other, the less used breast may become noticeably smaller. After weaning, the breasts will equal out in size.

If the baby suddenly refuses one breast, and you can feel a lump in it, this may indicate the possibility of a tumor. See a doctor for a thorough breast exam as soon as possible.

**Treatment measures for one-sided nursing**

1. Offer the baby her least favorite side first. After she has nursed on both sides, encourage her to nurse on the first side again.
2. Should the baby totally refuse one side, try changing positions. Use the football hold, or nurse while lying on your side. The baby may be more willing when she is sleepy or actually asleep, or when you nurse in a darkened room.
3. Increase the milk supply in the less used breast by manually expressing or pumping milk after each nursing for a few days.
4. If all else fails, simply accept your baby's preference to be a one-sided nurser.

## Sudden Refusal to Nurse

Occasionally a baby under six months suddenly refuses to nurse. A "nursing strike" usually lasts for a few days, but sometimes for as long as two weeks. It rarely means the baby is ready to wean. Weaning seldom occurs this suddenly. See Nursing Strike, Survival Guide for the Later Months, for the reasons behind this problem and suggestions for coping with it.

If your baby suddenly refuses one breast but is happy to nurse at the other, see One-Sided Nursing.

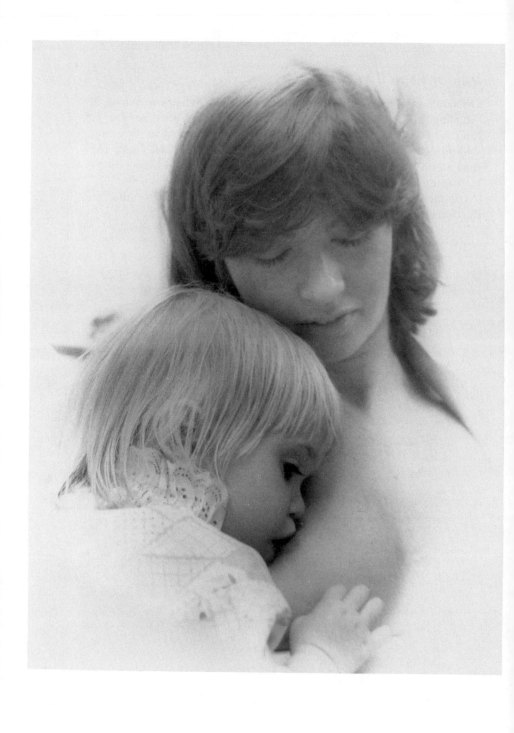

# CHAPTER SEVEN

# *Nursing the Older Baby and Toddler*

Nursing Your Six- to Twelve-Month-Old
The Transition to Table Food
Nursing Your Toddler
The Toddler's Diet
Nursing during Pregnancy
Tandem Nursing
Weaning

As BREASTFEEDING PROGRESSES PAST SIX MONTHS, THE NURSING RE-lationship continues to change. Although the baby is busy exploring the world around him and has shortened most of his feedings, breast milk continues to be his primary source of nutrients until he is well established on table foods. Breastfeeding also continues to provide protective antibodies against illness.

## Nursing Your Six- to Twelve-Month-Old

The typical baby of this age is venturing out on his own and seemingly becoming more independent, but he often scampers back to the safety and reassurance of his mother's arms. By eight to ten months, in fact, he probably cannot bear to have his mother out of his sight for even a minute. This is known as separation anxiety. Until the baby learns to trust that his mother will return, out of sight means gone forever.

It is during this time that many mothers experience a change in their babies' interest in nursing. One baby may become so intent on explor-ing that she has days when she is simply too busy to nurse. Another is more secure having his mother close by while he creeps about, turn-ing to her often for comfort and the breast. In either case, nursing now starts to become mainly a break for a snack and a bit of love and reassurance.

Many six- to eight-month-old babies, though not all, sleep until dawn. Night waking may be due to teething, separation anxiety, ill-ness, or a chill from kicking off the covers.

Many mothers notice that it takes longer for their milk to let down in these months. This may be a response to the lessening milk supply, and perhaps it is the reason some infants seem to lose interest in nurs-ing at around nine or ten months.

A woman's menstrual periods may return as the baby begins eating regular meals at the table. (Some women start menstruating earlier, however, and others do not until 12 to 18 months postpartum. Gener-ally, mothers who are nursing frequently find their periods resume much later.) These initial periods may be irregular. Some mothers re-port that their babies are fussy for a couple of days, or even refuse to nurse for a short time, when menstruation resumes. You may experi-ence sore nipples for one or two days during ovulation or just before starting your period.

You may sometimes feel tired and run-down during this time. Be-coming more active and getting overtired seems to be especially com-mon around six months postpartum. Certainly, eating poorly and los-ing too much weight can contribute to a loss of energy. Taking it a bit easier, getting some extra rest, and paying attention to your diet

can do a lot to improve your overall well-being. Taking a B-co
preparation may also be helpful.

## *The Transition to Table Food*

**From six to eight months.** Sometime after her sixth month, when your
baby is taking a total of a half cup of cereal in two feedings a day, she
is ready for other foods. She should still nurse before eating, however,
until she is well established on table foods and is having three meals
a day. The nutrients in breast milk are the ones that she needs most.

Because fruits and vegetables offer vitamins A and C, they become
important in the baby's diet as her intake of breast milk drops. They
also accustom her to different tastes and textures and encourage the
development of tongue control and chewing ability. Although puréed
fruits and vegetables, whether commercially prepared or homemade,
are nutritionally adequate, they do not accustom the baby to different
textures or help her learn chewing skills. Commercial baby food in
jars may be appropriate when you are eating out or traveling, but at
other times mashed soft fruits and vegetables are best.

The order in which fruits and vegetables are introduced isn't all that
important. Some nutritionists and others feel that vegetables may be
more readily accepted if they are introduced before fruits, whose
sweeter flavor many babies prefer. Fresh or canned fruits can be
mashed, scraped, diced, or chunked according to your baby's ability.
Fresh or frozen cooked vegetables are preferable to those that are
commercially canned, as these usually contain too much salt for a
baby. A food mill or baby-food grinder can be handy for vegetables
that are hard or stringy. Offer only one new food at a time, waiting
a few days before introducing another. In this way, should a certain
food upset the baby, you will have a good idea which one it is.

A meal pattern that works well during this transition time is cereal
and fruit in the morning and cereal and vegetables in the evening. Use
a fresh or frozen vegetable from your own dinner before it is salted or
seasoned.

Although one or two tablespoons of fruit is adequate, babies usually
like the taste so much they are eager for more. Limit the baby to one-
quarter or one-third cup per serving; too much fruit can cause intestinal upsets and diarrhea.

You can offer fruit juice instead, but limit the amount to three
ounces a day. "Juice abuse" is a common mistake in infant feeding.
Not only do babies not need more than three ounces, but juice often
lessens their appetite for milk and solid foods. Overdependence on

juice can lead to diarrhea and, especially when given in a bottle, to tooth decay. Avoid "fruit drinks," which contain mostly water, some juice, and sugar. Be careful with citrus, tomato, and pineapple juices—they can cause allergic reactions in some babies. Rashes, wheezing, nasal stuffiness, and diarrhea may be allergy symptoms. Juices bottled for infants are expensive and unnecessary. Once opened, fruit juices should not be stored in metal cans.

Juices are probably best offered from a cup. Most babies are ready to begin learning how to drink from a cup by the time they are seven or eight months old. At first you will need to hold the cup for the baby. Once he begins holding his own cup, be prepared for his turning the cup over to see what happens—all a part of the learning process. You can try a training cup, which comes with a tight-fitting lid and a spout and therefore won't spill; however, some babies suck from these, so the lesson goes unlearned.

One or two tablespoons of vegetable is sufficient for the baby. Vegetables high in nitrates, such as beets, carrots, and spinach, should be limited to this amount. When young infants are given excessive amounts of these vegetables, the nitrate can convert to nitrite in their bodies. This can cause the displacement of oxygen in the blood, leading to fast breathing and lethargy. *Methemoglobinemia*, as this condition is called, becomes less of a possibility after the baby is six months old and has more acid in her stomach.

Dark green and deep yellow vegetables, such as broccoli, carrots, sweet potatoes, and squash, should be given no more than three or four times a week. Given too often, they can cause the baby's skin to turn yellow. This is completely harmless, however.

During this time you can also offer the baby breads and dry cereals. These offer B vitamins and iron. Although the baby may not actually eat much as first, he will be developing his chewing and self-feeding skills. Rice cakes and dry Rice Chex or Corn Chex are good first choices before trying wheat-based breads and cereals. The chance of an allergic reaction to wheat lessens once the baby is seven or eight months old, but you may want to put off offering wheat even longer if anyone in the family is allergic to it.

Try not to worry should your baby eat very little before she is eight months old. She will have her own food preferences, and she may refuse a certain food one week and happily eat it the next. She may refuse all foods for a while if she is not feeling well. And, as she becomes interested in feeding herself, she may also turn her head at any food offered from a spoon. Although it is messy, you should let her feed herself. Give her another spoon, or allow her to use her fingers. Let her examine her food before deciding whether or not to eat it. By feeding herself, your baby will develop her grasping skills and hand-eye coordination. Be patient if she plays with her food instead of eating it; keep in mind that your breast milk is still the most important part of her diet.

**From eight to ten months.** Probably at some time between eight and ten months of age, your baby will become interested in what the rest of the family is eating. Again, I take my recommendations from Ellyn Satter and her wonderful guide to infant and toddler feeding, *Child of Mine: Feeding with Love and Good Sense* (1986).

Once table foods are offered, three major transitions follow. The first is adding another meal or two so the baby is eating three or four times a day. The second is adding high-protein foods—such as meat, poultry, fish, shell beans and lentils, eggs, cheese, tofu, and peanut butter—as the baby's intake of breast milk drops. The last transition is postponing breastfeeding until after the meal; this encourages the baby to take more solids.

This new meal pattern basically requires the addition of a midday meal and, perhaps, a small snack. Continuing to give a half cup of fortified infant cereal over one or two meals (or a meal and snack) is still important. Two servings of bread, at one-quarter slice a serving, complete the baby's requirement for grains. At least four daily servings of fruits and vegetables, at one to two tablespoons a serving, are recommended. Juice may substitute for one serving but should still be limited to three ounces a day.

The baby also needs at least two servings of high-protein foods every day. A serving of meat, poultry, fish, or eggs is about one tablespoon or one-half ounce. Although chicken and fish (carefully boned) are fairly easy for the baby to manage, red meats may need to be shredded, ground, or minced. Avoid lunch meats and hot dogs, which are high in salt and nitrates and are not the best sources of protein. The baby can have an egg three or four times a week. Should allergies be a concern, cook the egg until solid and offer only the yolk. Other high-protein foods for a baby of this age include: one ounce of hard cheese, one-quarter cup of cottage cheese, one-half cup of shell beans or lentils, and two tablespoons of peanut butter. Commercially prepared "infant dinners" are a poor source of protein, being mostly vegetables and water with only a small amount of meat.

Should you prefer that your child have a vegetarian diet, this is easy so long as cheese and eggs are included. Do take the time to learn all you can about vegetarianism and the nutritional needs of infants and toddlers; *Child of Mine* and *The New Laurel's Kitchen* (see Suggested Supplemental Reading) will get you started. You might also want to consult with a nutritionist, especially if you are considering a "vegan" (vegetable-only) diet. Young children on such diets are at substantial risk for B-vitamin deficiencies and, because of a lack of protein, general growth deficiencies. The federal Women, Infants, and Children (WIC) nutrition program or your local public health department can probably refer you to a nutritionist who can offer further guidance.

While your baby may not always get precisely the suggested amounts of grains, fruits, vegetables, and high-protein food every day, averaging close to these amounts over a week will ensure she is well nourished. But if by eight to ten months your baby will still take solids only sporadically at best, it may be time to give her a little extra encouragement. If her growth curve falls off, and, perhaps, she seems to be sick a lot, she may be becoming too emotionally dependent on the breast, and substituting nursing for eating a variety of nutritious foods. In this case, make sure you are nursing her after meals, not before. If she is desperate for the breast, try to keep the nursing short, then encourage her to return her attention to other foods. Always include her in family meals, but offer food at other times of the day if she refuses it at mealtimes. If she resents your pushing solids, have someone else feed her to let her feed herself. Never assume that because she spits something out in disgust one day she won't take it a week later.

**From ten to twelve months.** After the baby is established on table food, the final transition is adding milk along with the meal. Ideally this should be accomplished when the baby is between nine and twelve months of age. Whole milk is more digestible now that the baby is eating table foods. Low-fat milk is not a good choice because it does not provide the fat that the older baby or toddler needs. Evaporated milk, diluted one to one with water, can be used, however; this may be more convenient if your family routinely drinks low-fat milk. Because evaporated milk is treated with high heat, it is more digestible than whole milk. And it is no more expensive. You can use soy formula or another hypoallergenic formula if your baby is allergic to milk. If your baby does not like milk of any sort, offer plenty of cheese and yogurt, and try tofu—it is also very high in calcium.

You may be wondering right now if we have just weaned your baby. In a sense, yes. Weaning is the *process* of expanding your baby's diet to include other foods. For many of you, nursing will continue to be important and convenient for early morning feedings, snacks, naps, bedtime, and general soothing and comforting.

The baby's fluoride supplements should be stopped now if your water is fluoridated to 0.3 parts per million.

## *Nursing Your Toddler*

The toddler is trying to accomplish the major task of establishing himself as an individual. Although he is no longer a baby, he is still very dependent. One minute he is exploring and getting into everything, and the next he is turning to his mother for comfort and reassurance.

Many toddlers tend to nurse briefly. Some nurse just a few times a day, but many want the breast often. A toddler may nurse a few times one day, moreover, and many times the next. Even if he nurses infrequently, the antibodies in breast milk are still present and protective. The breast is important to the toddler not only for a quick snack and help in falling off to sleep, but for intermittent comfort and emotional refueling. Sometimes nursing is one of the toddler's few connections to a busy mother.

You may discover that nursing into toddlerhood is not only a convenient way of mothering, but that it is one of the few times during the day that your child holds still long enough for cuddling and affection.

Some nursing toddlers still wake at night for feedings. See the Survival Guide for the Later Months for suggestions and coping strategies.

The young toddler may be quite insistent when he wants to nurse, regardless of the time or place. As he gets a bit older he will become more willing to wait a little while.

Children in many parts of the world are breastfed until they are two, three, or four years of age, yet nursing a walking, talking toddler is considered somewhat deviant in parts of Western society. Many toddlers are dependent on a bottle, pacifier, thumb, or blanket, and this is quite accepted; but a mother who is nursing a toddler may have to deal with veiled or point-blank suggestions that her child is too old for it. The concerns about nursing beyond infancy often reflect the fear that a child will become spoiled or overdependent. In fact, when a toddler's need for security is met, he becomes more self-assured and independent.

Mothers who are nursing toddlers usually enjoy socializing with others who are doing the same. La Leche League is not only supportive of women who breastfeed beyond the first year, but also offers meetings for those who are nursing young children. Norma Jane Bumgarner's book *Mothering Your Nursing Toddler* (1982) is an excellent resource for those nursing beyond infancy.

## The Toddler's Diet

Toddlers are notorious as sporadic eaters. Their appetite decreases during this time—first because their growth slows down tremendously from that of the first year, and second because they are often too busy to eat. The toddler grows more in length than in weight. Weight gain typically slows to a pound or less every two months.

The toddler's feeding skills vary considerably. Sometimes she may feed herself, and other times she wants to be fed. Parents who worry about how little their child eats may be tempted to persuade, trick, or even force her to eat more. This turns meals into battles and may be the start of long-term feeding problems. As Ellyn Satter says, "You are responsible for *what* your child is offered to eat, *where* and *when* it is presented. She is responsible for *how much* of it she eats."

The suggested minimum servings of foods for the toddler are similar to those for the older baby. A handy rule of thumb is this: Give one tablespoon per year of age or one-quarter of the adult serving, which-ever is easiest to figure for the particular food. You would therefore offer your toddler two tablespoons of peas or one-quarter slice of apple. The suggested daily minimum servings for each food group are as follows:

- Fruits and vegetables: 4 servings
- Grains (bread, cereal, noodles, rice): 4 servings
- High-protein foods: 2 servings
- Milk: 2 to 3 cups

Offering a meal or nutritious snack every three to four hours is a good approach with a toddler. Don't always offer milk just because he likes it; if he drinks more than three cups a day it may replace other nutritious foods in his diet. Expect that your toddler may enjoy a certain food one day and refuse it the next. Make sure he comes to the table for meals and is offered whatever foods the family is eating. Do not play into his food whims by running out to the kitchen to fix something else for him when he refuses to eat.

## Nursing during Pregnancy

Although many people frown on breastfeeding during pregnancy, there is no reason you cannot continue nursing your child when you find out another is on the way. Fears that nursing will lead to miscar-riage or a malnourished newborn have no basis, even for mothers who are too queasy to eat much. Whether to wean is best left up to you—but if your nursing child is less than six months old, it may be desirable to at least delay weaning until he is eating solid foods and drinking from a cup.

Many women who nurse while pregnant complain of tender breasts and sore nipples. These are due to the hormonal changes of pregnancy. Many women also feel especially tired at first—this again is a normal response to pregnancy. Plenty of rest helps combat fatigue, especially in the first trimester. In the second and third trimesters, an excellent diet is essential for the nursing mother.

Pregnancy may cause decrease in the milk supply, and near the end the breasts revert to producing colostrum for the newborn. Some nursing babies and toddlers wean themselves at some point during their mothers' pregnancies. Others do not seem to mind the changes in the milk and show no signs of wanting to give up nursing.

## Tandem Nursing

Mothers who have nursed throughout all or most of their pregnancies may find themselves nursing an older baby or toddler along with the new baby. This may be overwhelming for some, particularly if the older child is nursing frequently. But many have found it to be a generally positive experience.

Because the breasts are receiving more stimulation than if the mother were nursing only one, the milk is usually plentiful. As a rule, the younger baby should be nursed first. Bumgarner's *Mothering Your Nursing Toddler* (1982) includes a detailed section on tandem nursing.

## Weaning

Ideally, complete weaning occurs when both the baby and the mother are ready for it. Weaning that is primarily initiated by the baby sometimes occurs before one year, but more commonly between two and four years.

Many times, though, a mother begins to think about weaning while her baby or toddler is still happily nursing. She may feel that weaning will make things easier—that it will put an end to night waking, make the baby more independent, or improve her own energy level. Some mothers have a self-imposed deadline for weaning and begin to feel pressured once it draws near. Others simply become fearful that their children will nurse forever. Most often, a mother considers weaning when other people suggest that the baby should no longer need to nurse. Criticism from friends, family, or health care workers may be straightforward or subtle, but it often motivates a mother to end the nursing relationship.

All mothers have mixed feelings about nursing at times. Keep in mind that weaning will not help your child sleep through the night, improve your relationship with your partner, make you less tired or less bored, or make the baby less dependent on you. Toddlers, especially, often demand to nurse more when their mothers become busier and when they receive little mothering except at the breast. At times that young children need more attention, ironically, mothers often feel most like they need some kind of a break. Weaning during these times can be terribly upsetting for a child, and for the rest of the family as well. Should the arbitrary date you had in mind for weaning arrive, there is no need to follow through if you and the baby are still enjoying nursing.

Everyone has her own opinion on how long a baby should nurse. Often this reflects her view of when a baby is no longer a baby. But there is no definite time at which your baby or toddler will no longer need to be nursed. Your child has her own timetable for achieving independence, and weaning will not speed the process. Mothers learn to deal with criticism in various ways, including keeping nursing a secret from certain people and telling others that they are weaning.

A mother might rightly initiate weaning if she has definite feelings against nursing a toddler or nursing while pregnant. Weaning—or simply limiting the number of daily feedings—may also be best when a mother is starting to resent nursing. The decision to wean should be made carefully, not in reaction to a bad day or a temporary problem.

Timing is important once the decision to wean has been reached. Although it is generally easier to wean before a child is 18 months old, keep in mind that weaning is a process rather than an event. Abrupt weaning can be devastating for a child. Weaning initiated by the mother should occur gradually and empathetically over several weeks at least. There are also better times than others to initiate the process. If the child is particularly clingy and needy, if she has recently had a stressful experience such as moving or starting child care, or if you are actively trying to get her to sleep through the night, now is not the time to wean.

Specific suggestions for weaning can be found in the Survival Guide for the Later Months. In general, mother-led weaning involves substituting for nursing something that the child enjoys as much. In this way weaning does not become a series of deprivations or rejections. If the pace of weaning is too rapid, most children will react with obvious unhappiness or increased dependency on a pacifier, a thumb, or a bottle. Occasionally weaning must be postponed for a few weeks because the child is simply unable to cope without nursing.

Whether weaning is initiated by the mother or is a mutual undertaking, feelings of sadness are bound to arise as the final days arrive, marking the end of the precious months spent together nursing. Once the nursings become infrequent, the breasts may look smaller and feel less firm. Most women can express milk for several months after nursing has stopped. The breasts typically regain their former size and shape within six months of weaning.

# SURVIVAL GUIDE
## for the Later Months

Night Waking
Nursing Strike
Weaning the Older Baby (Eight to Twelve Months)
Weaning the Toddler

## Night Waking

Although most older babies and toddlers sleep six or more hours at a stretch, some wake up night after night. Whether teething, separation anxiety, or loneliness causes night waking, authorities on child development recommend one of two ways of dealing with it. Some believe that the child should be comforted and nursed back to sleep. The rest feel the persistent waker should be taught to sleep through the night. The two camps generally agree that weaning or offering a late evening feeding rarely helps a child sleep through the night.

You can find encouragement for accepting your child's wakefulness in books such as Tine Thevenin's *The Family Bed: An Age Old Concept in Child Rearing* (1976) and Norma Jane Bumgarner's *Mothering Your Nursing Toddler* (1982). Many parents find that simply allowing the baby to nurse and sleep in their bed is least disruptive. Some have come up with other arrangements such as adjusting the crib to the side of the bed so the baby can easily be moved back and forth, or placing a mattress on the floor for night nursing.

A couple may feel that their older baby is ready to master the task of settling himself back to sleep at night. Getting him to do so involves putting him in his own bed and, when he cries, reassuring him without picking him up. Practically speaking, the child simply cries it out for a few nights. Although this may seem drastic, many parents report that it works.

If you decide to try this strategy, make plans with your partner, selecting a three- to four-day period in advance. When the time comes, go to your crying baby every five minutes; lay him down; say, "It's night-night time," and leave. Most babies cry up to an hour or so the first night, and for a shorter time the next two or three nights.

Here are some other suggestions, which come without guarantees: Double-diaper the child with rubber pants, or put him in disposable diapers, to avoid night changes. Make sure he is warm or cool enough at night by using pajamas with feet or a sleeping bag in cold weather, or a fan when it is hot. Sometimes fathers can lull a child back to sleep by rocking or offering something to drink from a cup. You'll want to talk the problem over with your partner and develop a plan together.

## Nursing Strike

Although nursing strikes can occur at any time, they usually happen in the second half of the baby's first year. A nursing strike is distinguished from weaning by its suddenness. Some babies wean themselves between eight and twelve months, but they usually do so gradually.

Reasons for nursing strikes vary greatly. They may include teething, a cold, an ear infection, a painful herpes sore in the mouth, or a change in the taste of the milk. They sometimes happen after a prolonged separation between a baby and her mother, or after a baby has bitten her mother and been frightened by her response. Sometimes, when a baby has become used to a bottle and its rapid flow of milk, her refusal to nurse is a response to her mother's dwindling milk supply. Some authorities believe a nursing strike may precede mastery of a major motor skill, such as crawling, standing, or walking.

Although some mothers decide to turn a nursing strike into final weaning, in most cases the baby can be coaxed to resume nursing. Strikes typically last a few days but may go on for as long as two weeks.

**Treatment measures for nursing strikes**

1. Try a change in position, or nurse in a quiet, darkened room.
2. So long as the baby refuses to nurse, pump or manually express your milk frequently throughout the day. Offer the milk in a cup rather than a bottle.
3. Try to determine the cause for the nursing strike. Consider having the baby examined to rule out an ear infection or other physical problem. Check your milk supply, especially if the baby has been nursing infrequently or has become increasingly dependent on a bottle: Do your breasts feel empty most of the time? Is the milk slow to let down? Is the baby swallowing less?
4. Maintain frequent and close skin-to-skin contact with the baby without nursing. Offer the breast whenever the baby is sleepy.

## Weaning the Older Baby (Eight to Twelve Months)

Weaning the older baby need not be hard, especially if he is crawling and busily exploring or has lost interest in some of his nursings. Ideally, weaning at any age should occur gradually, over several weeks at least. A good place to begin is with the nursing that the baby seems least interested in, most likely one during the day. Key to your success is providing an appealing substitute for the breast. This means offering not only something else to eat or drink, but also yourself. Nursing provides a mother's love and attention as well as food. You'll need to do a lot of cuddling and rocking, and activities like reading a book or playing on the floor together.

You must choose whether to wean to a cup or a bottle. Although the older baby is developmentally ready for a cup, if he has trouble swallowing from one, the bottle may be best. However, giving the baby a bottle can lead to other difficulties. If he is not carefully monitored, he can become overdependent on the bottle, lose interest in solid foods, and end up with serious tooth decay. If you wean the baby to a bottle, of course, you will probably need to wean him *from* it later on.

Unless the baby is well established on table foods and eating three meals a day, give formula or evaporated milk diluted one to one with water before offering solid foods.

Although weaning may progress quickly for some babies, concluding in a month or two, other babies take longer, especially those who are especially fond of nursing or are reluctant to give up certain feedings. The first nursing in the morning and those before nap time and bedtime are often most loved by the older baby. It may take longer to eliminate these completely.

## Weaning the Toddler

Although the weaning process is similar at all ages, the toddler is often especially attached to the breast and deserves extra consideration. Weaning a toddler involves a good deal of time and attention.

Unfortunately, no one technique works for every mother and toddler. The best recommendations involve finding substitutions and distractions that may satisfy the child, while at the same time ensuring that her needs for food, love, and attention are met. No plan is likely to succeed, however, unless a mother is sure of her desire to wean. Her attitude is most important to her success.

Before you begin, pay close attention to the baby's nursing routine, and yours. Keeping a record for a few days, like the one below, may give you some valuable insights for developing an effective plan.

| Time | Place | Interest level | Reason for nursing |
| --- | --- | --- | --- |

Take note of when and where you nurse, the baby's level of interest in nursing, and what you think prompted her demand for the breast. From the toddler's point of view, nursing may be just the thing whenever she is bored, frustrated or tired, or wants your attention or comfort—as well as when she is hungry.

From your observations, you should be able to identify which nursings are least crucial to your toddler and get some clues as to what type of substitutions will most likely satisfy. Some nursings may be easily replaced with a nutritious snack or something to drink. Substitutions for toddlers may include any number of activities—playing with a special toy, reading a book, taking a walk, or visiting with

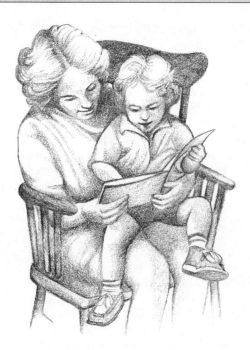

another toddler. Warm weather months may be an easier time to encourage weaning, as most toddlers enjoy exploring out of doors.

Although you may be able to substitute certain predictable daily
nursings with other activities, if your toddler nurses sporadically all
day you may sometimes need to coax her to postpone nursings. Delaying daytime nursings works well for some toddlers as long as some
distraction is provided. This can be an effective way to further
weaning.

Some of your nursings are probably associated with routines the
two of you have established, and with recurrent situations in which
your toddler wants to nurse to get your attention. Identify these instances so you can change the pattern. If you nurse in bed early in the
morning get up instead—get dressed and offer your child breakfast. If
you have a favorite place to relax and nurse, stay away from it. If
your toddler demands to nurse every time you talk on the phone, keep
conversations short. If you sit in front of the television and nurse, do
something else or she will want to continue with the usual pattern.
Think creatively of ways your child can learn new routines.

You can also take advantage of your child's ability to understand
language. Talk to her about nursing—especially if you are trying to
postpone feedings. She may accept your wish to "save up the milk till
nap time and night-night." Older toddlers may be able to agree to

future weaning upon an upcoming birthday or other milestone, such as the start of preschool.

The bedtime nursing may continue as the child's favorite. Some mothers find this is a special time for themselves as well, and continue with it for weeks or months after other feedings have been abandoned. If you want to wean the baby completely, your partner or another family member may be able to help the child establish a non-nursing bedtime routine.

# Resources for Nursing Mothers

## Breastfeeding Support and Education

La Leche League International
9616 Minneapolis Avenue
Franklin Park, Illinois 60131
800-LA LECHE

Call between 9:00 A.M. and 3:00 P.M.
CST for breastfeeding help or a referral to a local La Leche group.

Boston Association for Childbirth
  Education (BACE)
Nursing Mothers' Council
184 Savin Hill Avenue
Dorchester, Massachusetts 02125
617-244-5102

Childbirth Education Association of
  Greater Philadelphia
Nursing Mothers' Support Groups
5 East Second Avenue
Conshohocken, Pennsylvania 19428
215-828-0131

Nursing Mothers Counsel, Inc.
P.O. Box 50063
Palo Alto, California 94303
415-591-6688

Nursing Mothers Counsel has chapters in various cities in California; in Denver, Colorado; in Ft. Wayne, Indiana; and in Atlanta, Georgia. Call for a local number.

International Lactation Consultant
  Association
P.O. Box 4031
University of Virginia Station
Charlottesville, Virginia 22903

## Electric Breast Pump Rental

Call toll free for the address of the station nearest you.

Medela, Inc.
P.O. Box 386
Crystal Lake, Illinois 60014
800-435-8316
(From Illinois, Alaska, or Hawaii call
  collect 815-455-6920)

Egnell, Inc.
765 Industrial Drive
Cary, Illinois 60013
800-323-8750
(From Illinois, Alaska, or Hawaii call
  collect 312-639-2900)

## Breast Shells

Breast shells are available by mail order from Nurse-Dri and by phone or mail order from Medela.

*Nurse-Dri Breast Shields: $11.95 (includes shipping)*
Nurse-Dri Breast Shield Co.
P.O. Box 541
Corte Madera, California 94925
415-332-1616

*Medela Breast Shields: $11.95 plus shipping*
Medela, Inc.
P.O. Box 386
Crystal Lake, Illinois 60014
800-435-8316
(From Illinois, Alaska, or Hawaii call collect 815-455-6920)

## Breast Milk Cooler

This canvas-covered styrofoam cooler for storing and transporting breast milk contains refreezable ice packs and three bottles. Order the Medela Canvas Cooler Case for $39.95 (plus shipping) from—

Medela, Inc.
P.O. Box 386
Crystal Lake, Illinois 60014
800-435-8316
(From Illinois, Alaska, or Hawaii call
    collect 815-455-6920)

## Nursing Supplementation Devices

A nursing supplementation device provides supplementary milk or formula while a baby is being breastfed. Such a device may be used in a variety of situations, most commonly when the baby is adopted or the mother wishes to relactate after a period of not nursing. It may also be used when the mother wishes to build up or supplement a low milk supply, the baby is slow to gain weight, or the baby has a cleft palate, a cardiac disorder, or a weak or ineffective suck.

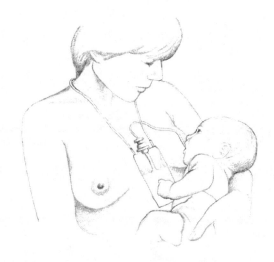

A supplementation device usually consists of a plastic pouch to hold milk or formula and a thin, flexible tube that is placed on top of the mother's breast and ends at the nipple. As the baby nurses, he receives the supplement along with whatever milk his mother is producing. These devices should be used with the guidance of an experienced lactation professional. Currently, they can be ordered from—

*Lact-Aid: about $33.00 plus shipping*
Lact-Aid International
P.O. Box 1066
Athens, Tennessee 37303
800-228-1933
(From Tennessee call 615-744-9090)

*Supplemental Nutrition System: $33.25 plus shipping*
Medela, Inc.
P.O. Box 386
Crystal Lake, Illinois 60014
800-435-8316
(From Illinois, Alaska, or Hawaii call collect 815-455-6920)

The devices may also be available in your area through a local lactation professional. Lact-Aid and Medela will be happy to refer you to a local source.

## Nursing Pillow

The Nurse Mate nursing pillow circles the mother's waist to help position a baby more comfortably. It is ideal for nursing twins simultaneously. The pillow costs $35.95 plus $4.50 for shipping and handling. You can order it by mail or phone from—

Four Dee Products
Dept. NMC
6014 Lattimer
Houston, Texas 77035
713-728-0389

# The Safety of Drugs during Breastfeeding
*By Philip O. Anderson, Pharm. D.*

If you are considering taking a drug while nursing, you are likely wondering what effects it may have on your baby and on milk production. Clear guidelines are hard to come by in this situation. This appendix will explain what you should consider before taking a particular drug, and how, if you take it, you can minimize its effects on your child.

## The Excretion of Drugs into Milk

Almost any drug you take will reach your milk in some quantity. Although you would never want to expose your baby to a foreign chemical unnecessarily, the amount of drug that appears in milk is often not great enough to harm a nursing child. Several considerations are important when deciding whether to take a particular drug.

**Your baby's age and maturity.** Just as your baby becomes better able to move about as he grows older, his ability to metabolize and detoxify foreign chemicals and drugs improves with time. Premature infants have little capacity for metabolizing drugs; when a premie needs treatment for a medical condition, drugs are often given in much smaller doses than they would be for a full-term newborn or an older infant. The amount of medication in a mother's milk that is safe for a one-month-old, therefore, may be considered dangerous for a premature infant. Likewise, a baby who is several months old has a much greater capacity to handle drugs in breast milk than does a one-month-old.

**Your needs.** Maybe you have a serious medical condition that threatens your health and your ability to care for your child, and you must take medication for it. But maybe you're suffering from only a minor discomfort, and can get by without drugs. Whatever your condition, you must evaluate its seriousness and the consequences of not taking a particular drug. Then weigh these consequences against the benefits of breastfeeding, as you see them. You may decide to pump your milk and discard it for the period you will need the medication or, if necessary, give up nursing altogether rather than expose your baby to a potentially hazardous drug.

**The duration of treatment.** If you have a chronic health problem, such as high blood pressure, you may be taking a drug over a long period. But maybe you need medication for only a few days, as with many antibiotics, or even just once, as with an anesthetic for a dental procedure or a diagnostic agent for an X-ray. If only brief drug therapy is needed, you can avoid exposing your infant to harmful amounts of the drug while not completely giving up breast-feeding.

**The history of the drug.** If a drug has been used for many years—especially if it has been given frequently to infants or to nursing mothers—it is possible to predict with confidence the risks it poses to the breastfed baby. This is not so, however, for a drug that is new on the market, or one that has never been used in children or infants. With no "track record" to go on, health care providers will vary in their assessments of the risks your baby faces from small amounts of the drug in your milk. You may get different advice from different physicians—your obstetrician and the baby's pediatrician, for example.

**The persistence of the drug in the body.** Some drugs are eliminated from the body after only a few hours, whereas others remain a long time and "accumu-late." Accumulation is measured by the "half-life" of the drug; it takes four to five half-lives for a drug to be eliminated from the body. "Long-acting" drugs, or those with long half-lives, are more likely to persist in milk and be present at the time of breastfeeding than "short-acting" drugs, those with short half-lives. Long-acting drugs are also more likely to accumulate in the baby and affect her health.

**Coordinating feedings and dosage.** If a drug is short-acting, or quickly elimi-nated, you may be able to time the doses in a way that will minimize the amount of drug in your milk at feedings. You might take a dose just after nursing, so the amount of drug in the milk peaks between feedings. If you are on a once-a-day medication, you might take it after the last feeding of the evening and substitute milk expressed during the day or formula later in the night; by morning the amount of drug in your milk may be down to an accept-ably low level. These strategies work best with older infants who are nursing at infrequent intervals.

These techniques work in part because drugs pass in both directions be-tween your bloodstream and breast milk. As the drug levels in your blood-stream decrease, the drug in your milk will pass back into your bloodstream. When breastfeeding must be withheld because of drug therapy that may harm an infant, expressing milk is sometimes advocated in the mistaken belief that the drug will thereby be eliminated from the milk sooner. Because of the re-verse passage of drugs from milk to the bloodstream and because only a very small fraction of the drug in your body is in your milk, pumping your breasts and discarding the milk ("pumping and dumping") has very little effect on the eventual amount of drug your baby gets from your milk. Pumping the breasts may be useful, though, in maintaining your milk supply and decreasing any pain from engorgement during temporary discontinuation of breast-feeding.

**Route of administration.** The way that you take a medication helps determine how much of the drug will get into your bloodstream and to your baby. Drugs given by injection go directly into your bloodstream and have access to the milk, but some injected drugs cannot be absorbed into the infant's bloodstream from his gastrointestinal tract. Medications given by mouth usually appear in your bloodstream, except for some that are meant to work locally in the stomach or intestines. Significant amounts of drugs can be absorbed from drops and ointments placed in the eye. Vaginal and rectal products can be absorbed into the bloodstream. The amount of a drug that reaches your bloodstream is usually less if taken by an inhaler than if taken by mouth. Creams and ointments that are applied to your skin usually do not allow very much drug into your bloodstream and are generally safe to use while nursing. Be careful, though, not to get the ointment or cream on your baby's skin or allow him to get any into his mouth.

## The Effects of Drugs on Lactation

Not only may the drugs you take affect your baby directly, but they can potentially influence your milk production. This could happen in a number of ways, since several hormones work together to control lactation. Some drugs are used deliberately to stimulate or stop milk flow; however, a few medications intended for another purpose have been shown to affect lactation. Those that have are identified in this appendix.

## Common Drugs and Their Safety

In the following list, common drugs are grouped into categories and subcategories according to their uses. Their potential effects on the breastfeeding infant and, where applicable, on lactation itself are noted. Drug names that begin with a lower-case letter are generic; those that begin with a capital letter are brand names. A more complete listing of brand names is in the Index to Common Drugs at the end of this appendix.

**Acne products.** If applied only to the face, topical *tretinoin* is safe to use. Other topical products such as *benzoyl peroxide, clindamycin* or *erythromycin* are safe to use. *Isotretinoin*, which is given by mouth, should not be used while nursing. Daily long-term use of *tetracycline* for acne is not desirable while nursing.

**Anesthetics.**

*General Anesthetics. Nitrous oxide* is sometimes used for dental procedures. By the time you no longer feel its effects (usually within an hour), it is safe to resume nursing. General anesthetics used in hospitals for major operations have not been studied with nursing and generally persist in the body longer than nitrous oxide. Consult your anesthesiologist before the operation to see when you can resume nursing.

*Local Anesthetics.* These drugs are given by injection for dental or other short procedures. Information on their effects during nursing is available for only two drugs, *lidocaine* and *bupivicaine.* Both of these drugs are safe to use while nursing. With other local anesthetics, breastfeeding should be withheld for six to eight hours after the procedure as a precaution.

**Anti-infective agents.** Most drugs that are taken for infections reach the milk in only small quantities—too small to treat the same infections in an infant. Occasionally, though, these small amounts can disrupt the normal balance of microorganisms in the baby's mouth and intestines. This may result in thrush, an overgrowth of yeast in the mouth, (see Thrush Nipples, Survival Guide for the First Week, and Fussiness and Colic, Survival Guide for the First Two Months), or in diarrhea or diaper rash, caused by an overgrowth of yeast or other organisms in the bowel. Although neither condition is generally serious, and both can be readily treated, it is important to watch for their signs while you are taking antibacterials. The likelihood of thrush or diarrhea occurring depends on the particular drug you are taking. Some antibacterials may cause other problems, as noted.

*Acyclovir.* This antiviral drug reaches fairly high levels in milk when given orally or by intravenous injection. Breastfeeding is not recommended while using acyclovir by these routes. Use of topical acyclovir ointment poses little threat to the infant.

*Penicillins.* These are very safe drugs that are often given directly to infants as treatment for infections. Occasionally allergies develop to penicillins, so the baby should be watched for rashes. If you see signs of rash, thrush, or diarrhea, call the health care provider.

*Cephalosporins.* These are similar to penicillins, and the same precautions apply. Some of the newer, more potent cephalosporins given by injection are more likely to cause thrush and diarrhea.

*Erythromycin.* This is a very safe drug that is often given directly to infants. It poses no unusual problems when taken by a nursing mother. See also Acne products.

*Furazolidone.* This drug is known to be poorly absorbed into the bloodstream after oral use. It is safe to use while nursing; it may be given safely to infants over one month of age. It is an alternative to metronidazole for *Giardia* infections if the infant is over one month old.

*Quinolones.* Newer quinolones such as *norfloxacin* and *ciprofloxacin* have not been well studied in nursing infants and are not given directly to infants or children. It is best to avoid these drugs if possible or to withhold breastfeeding while they are used.

*Sulfonamides (sulfas).* Large doses given directly to newborn infants can increase the risk of jaundice (yellowing of the skin and eyes). Other medications are usually preferred if the baby is premature or if the sulfonamide is long-acting; watch for rashes as well as jaundice.

*Septra* and *Bactrim* are common drugs that contain a moderately long-acting sulfonamide. Because little is known about the excretion of these drugs into milk, alternatives should be considered if the baby is less than one month old. The same precaution pertains to *sulfamethoxazole (Gantanol)*. *Sulfisoxazole (Gantrisin)* appears in milk in only very small amounts and seems safe to use while nursing. Combination tablets containing the red dye phenazopyridine *(Pyridium)*, such as *Azo-Gantrisin* or *Azo-Gantanol*, should be avoided, particularly with newborns.

*Tetracyclines.* These should generally not be given to children because they cause staining of the teeth. The amounts that appear in milk, however, are very small and are somewhat inactivated by the calcium in milk. Tetracyclines can probably be used safely by the nursing mother for short periods if no other drug is available. See also Acne products.

*Nitrofurantoin.* This appears in small amounts in breast milk; these amounts are generally not harmful to infants over one month of age.

*Metronidazole.* In the treatment of *Trichomonas* infections, this drug can be given as a single 1- to 2-gram dose. Breastfeeding should be stopped temporarily, but can be resumed 24 hours after the (last) dose.

*Chloramphenicol.* It is best to avoid this drug during nursing; mothers who have used it report fussiness during feeding and refusal of the breast. Additionally, there is a small possibility of its causing serious blood disorders in the infant. If the drug is essential, breastfeeding should be stopped, at least temporarily.

*Aminoglycosides.* These drugs are given primarily in the hospital, by injection. Amounts in milk are very small and pose no danger to the breastfed infant.

*Isoniazid.* This drug, used to treat tuberculosis, enters the milk in very small amounts. It poses a slight risk of damage to the baby's liver. If needed, however, it is safer to treat the mother with the drug than to risk exposing the infant to tuberculosis. Watch the infant for signs of jaundice.

**Scabicides and pediculocides.** These drugs are used to treat scabies, a skin condition caused by mites, and pediculosis, or infestation with lice. The most common medication, *lindane (Kwell)*, is very fat-soluble and can persist in milk and in the baby's body a long time, particularly when used in excessive amounts or too frequently. While no harm has been reported in breastfed infants due to lindane, there are a number of safe alternative treatments. For lice, *synergized pyrethrins (Rid* and *A-200*, for example) can be used, and for scabies, *permethrin (Elimite)* is a related, safe alternative.

**Pain and arthritis medications.**

*Acetaminophen.* This drug is safe to use during lactation.

*Aspirin.* It is safe to use aspirin occasionally, but take it just after nursing, or at least one to two hours before the next feeding. When large doses are taken daily, as for arthritis, problems can sometimes occur; consult your health care provider.

*Nonsteroidal anti-inflammatory agents. Ibuprofen, naproxen,* and *diclofenac* appear in only minute amounts in the milk; they seem safe to use during lactation. Some of the older, more toxic agents in this group, such as *indomethacin* and *phenylbutazone,* should be avoided during breastfeeding. Many of the newer drugs in the class, such as *sulindac, tolmetin, piroxicam,* and *diflunisal,* have not been well studied in breastfed infants. They should be avoided if possible.

*Narcotics.* When used in normal amounts for pain relief, narcotics—including *codeine, hydrocodone, propoxyphene, Percocet, Percodan,* and even injections of *morphine* and *meperidine*—pose no hazard to the breastfed infant. Narcotic addicts, however, can addict their infants through the milk. Methadone maintenance for narcotic addiction can be carefully undertaken during breastfeeding, with close supervision by a health care provider.

**Ergot alkaloids.**

*Ergotamine.* This is a component of several products, such as *Cafergot,* used in the treatment of migraine. Some ergot alkaloids have been found to cause vomiting in breastfed infants whose mothers have taken the drugs. While ergotamine itself has not been studied, it seems prudent to avoid it while breastfeeding.

*Other ergot drugs. Ergonovine (Ergotrate)* and *methylergonovine (Methergine)* are often given to mothers right after delivery to diminish uterine bleeding. With the usual doses and the normal length of treatment, these drugs cause no problems in the breastfed infant. Large amounts, however, can cause nausea, vomiting, and diarrhea in the baby. These effects have been said to occur occasionally when the drugs are used beyond the immediate postpartum period.

**Immunosuppressive agents.** This group includes the drugs used to treat cancer, medications for severe arthritis and certain skin diseases, and drugs administered after organ transplantation. Because these agents are among the most toxic used in medicine, very few women have breastfed while taking them. Little is known about their passage into milk, therefore, but even small amounts, should they reach the baby, could cause harm. Because these drugs are used for only very severe conditions, it is usually more important for the mother to take the drug than it is for her to nurse her baby. Hence, breastfeeding should not be undertaken, except possibly during treatment with *azathio-*

*prine (Imuran)* following organ transplantation. A few mothers have safely breastfed their infants while taking this drug after kidney transplant. This should be attempted, however, only after consultation with the physician. *Cyclosporine* is frequently used as an immunosuppresant following organ transplantation, but has not been well studied in nursing. Preliminary study shows that it is probably not safe to nurse while taking this drug.

**Anticoagulants.** Anticoagulants are rarely taken by breastfeeding women, but occasionally their use is necessary. They can be of the injectable type (such as *heparin*) or of the oral type (such as *warfarin*). Heparin can be safely used during lactation because it does not pass into milk. Although warfarin *(Coumadin)* has been thought for many years to endanger the breastfeeding infant, more recent evidence indicates that it is probably safe to use as well. This is not true for other oral anticoagulants, many of which have caused bleeding in breastfed infants.

**Anticonvulsants.** Anticonvulsants are used to treat epilepsy and other seizure disorders. Because these medications are used continuously and are often long-acting, they should be taken with caution during breastfeeding. The baby may show no effects other than subtle behavioral changes, so be vigilant.

*Phenobarbital.* This drug has been used in infants for many years with no severe adverse effects. You can use it safely during breastfeeding, although it may make the baby drowsy and less interested in nursing.

*Phenytoin.* This drug has been used for many years by breastfeeding women. It appears to be safe.

*Primidone.* This is similar to phenobarbital; the same precautions apply.

*Carbamazepine.* This drug, as well as its active metabolite, is known to pass into milk in significant amounts. Although no adverse effects in infants have been reported, the excretion of significant amounts of the drug into milk is a reason for caution.

*Valproic acid.* Only very small amounts of this drug enter milk; however, the drug can cause severe, though rare, liver damage. The infant should be watched carefully, particularly for signs of jaundice.

*Other anticonvulsants.* These have not been well studied in breastfeeding women and their infants. Be particularly cautious if you are nursing while taking them.

**Cough, cold, allergy, and asthma medications.** The various drugs used for these conditions of the respiratory tract are often used together in combination products. These are best avoided during breastfeeding. Usually only one symptom is really troublesome, and a single-ingredient product can treat it effectively. For example, hay fever and allergies can be treated with an antihistamine alone, and a cough can be treated with a single-ingredient cough syrup.

198 Appendix B: The Safety of Drugs during Breastfeeding

Drugs taken as nasal sprays or by inhaler generally reach the milk in lesser quantities than those taken orally. Sustained-release products should be avoided. Common sore throat lozenges *(Sucrets, Chloraseptic)* are safe to use.

*Antihistamines.* Antihistamines are used in many products for allergy, colds, coughs, and inducing sleep. They can reach the infant through breast milk in amounts large enough to cause drowsiness. High doses of antihistamines can theoretically decrease milk flow, particularly in combination with decongestants, so use no more than necessary to control symptoms. Often a single dose at bedtime is sufficient. If you are planning to use an oral product, choose one with 2 milligrams or less of *chlorpheniramine, brompheniramine, dexchlorpheniramine,* or *dexbrompheniramine* per dose, or 25 milligrams or less of *diphenhydramine* per dose, and avoid sustained-release products.

*Decongestants.* These drugs might cause agitation or fussiness in an infant, but little is known about their passage into milk. Decongestants can decrease milk flow, so use no more than necessary to control symptoms. Nasal sprays *(Afrin, Nostrilla)* are preferable to oral drugs; if you are planning to use an oral product, choose one with 30 milligrams or less of *ephedrine, pseudoephedrine,* or *phenylpropanolamine* per dose, avoid sustained-release products, and be aware of a possible decrease in milk supply.

*Theophylline.* *Aminophylline* and other theophylline products have been well studied in breast milk. Occasionally they can cause jitteriness and agitation in infants, usually newborns. In general, though, they are safe.

*Cough medicines.* The two common drugs are *guaiafenesin* and *dextromethorphan,* both of which are safe to use during breastfeeding. Rarely, iodide drugs such as *potassium iodide (SSKI)* or *iodinated glycerol (Organidin)* are prescribed as expectorants. Iodine becomes concentrated in milk and subsequently in the infant's thyroid gland; iodide rashes have also occurred in breastfed infants. Iodides should not be used during lactation.

**Heart and blood pressure drugs.** These drugs are rarely used in women of breastfeeding age, and information about them is therefore limited. Very little is known, in particular, about newer agents in the group.

*ACE inhibitors.* *Captopril* and *enalapril* may be safe to use while nursing, but there is only limited experience with them.

*Beta blockers.* The oldest drug in the group, *propranolol,* is also the best studied and safest. *Metoprolol* and *labetalol* also appear safe to use. These drugs reach the milk in insignificant amounts.

Some of the newer, long-acting drugs such as *nadolol, atenolol, timolol,* and *acebutolol* reach the milk in higher quantities, and are also more likely to accumulate in the infant's bloodstream. These should be avoided during breastfeeding, especially with a newborn.

*Calcium channel blockers.* Information on *diltiazem, nifedipine,* and *verapamil* is limited, but amounts in milk do not appear to be large enough to affect nursing infants.

*Digoxin.* This drug is excreted into milk in only small amounts, and is therefore safe to use during breastfeeding.

*Hydralazine.* Amounts of this drug excreted into milk are small. It can be used safely during lactation.

*Methyldopa.* Amounts of this drug excreted into milk are small. It can also be used safely during lactation.

*Reserpine.* This drug can cause nasal stuffiness in infants and should be avoided during lactation.

*Procainamide.* Amounts that reach the milk are small. This drug appears safe to use while nursing.

**Diuretics.** Large doses of diuretics, especially the most potent ones and those that are long-acting, can decrease milk production; diuretics have been used therapeutically for this purpose. Passage into milk has not been well studied, but small amounts might be expected to cause rashes or other allergic phenomena in infants on rare occasions.

*Furosemide.* This is a potent drug that has been used to suppress lactation. It should be used cautiously in small doses.

*Hydrochlorothiazide.* In usual doses given once daily, this drug appears safe. Larger doses given several times daily could suppress lactation.

*Other thiazides.* Long-acting thiazides should be avoided during breast-feeding.

*Chlorthalidone.* This is a very long-acting agent that should not be used during breastfeeding because it suppresses lactation. It also accumulates in the infant.

*Spironolactone.* This drug and its metabolite appear in significant amounts in milk.

**Gastrointestinal drugs.** Many of the drugs in this class act locally in the stomach and intestine and are not absorbed into the bloodstream; they cannot, therefore, appear in milk. Other gastrointestinal drugs *are* absorbed, and can affect the infant through breast milk. If a choice exists, it is prudent to choose a drug that is not absorbable.

*Antidiarrheals.* Bulk-forming fibers *(Metamucil, Fibercon)* and kaolin and pectin mixtures *(Kao-Pectate)* are not absorbed and can be used safely to firm up loose or watery stools. *Bisthmuth subsalicylate (Pepto-Bismol)* is best avoided because of the large amount of salicylate it contains. *Loperamide* and *diphenoxylate* have not been well studied and should be used sparingly and with caution while nursing.

*Nonabsorbable laxatives.* Bulk-forming laxatives such as bran and other fibers *(Metamucil, Fibercon)* are not absorbed into the bloodstream and are therefore safe. Likewise, stool softening agents such as *docusate (Colace)* are not absorbable. Saline cathartics such as *Phospho-Soda* and *milk of magnesia* are poorly absorbed and do not affect the composition of milk.

*Absorbable cathartics.* Many of the more potent laxatives are absorbed into the bloodstream and have caused increased frequency of stools in breastfed infants. Laxatives in this class include *cascara* and *danthron.* *Aloe* and *senna* can affect the breastfed infant if taken in high doses, but are safe to use occasionally in small amounts.

*Antacids.* These are poorly absorbed and are safe to use during breastfeeding.

*Histamine H-2 antagonists.* *Cimetidine* and *ranitidine* both reach high levels in breast milk and are best avoided. The newer drugs, *famotidine* and *nizatidine* have not been studied, but are probably quite similar. In older infants who are not nursing at night, a single daily dose at bedtime after the baby's last feeding can be used. *Sucralfate* (see below) is an alternative.

*Sucralfate.* This locally acting drug poses no harm to the breastfed infant.

**Hormones.** There are a number of classes of drugs that fall into the category of hormones, and each must be considered separately. Because hormones are potent agents that can affect the development of the infant, it is of paramount importance to consider both the dosage and the duration of therapy.

*Corticosteriods.* Drugs in this category include *cortisone, prednisone,* and *dexamethasone.* Low doses and short courses of therapy (one to two weeks) appear to pose no harm to the infant. Of concern are long courses of treatment (several weeks to months) with moderate to large doses. Although only a small fraction of each dose appears in milk, it is unknown what these amounts will do to the developing infant.

*Corticosteroid inhalers* for asthma or nasal allergies pose less of a threat because the doses are small. Many of the systemic effects of these drugs are due to swallowed drug that is absorbed into the bloodstream from the intestine. To minimize the baby's exposure, rinse your mouth and throat after using the inhaler and avoid swallowing any excess. These drugs include *beclomethasone, flunisolide,* and the inhaler forms of *triamcinolone.*

*Oral contraceptives.* Taking "the pill" is the least desirable method of birth control during breastfeeding. The hormones in oral contraceptives are potent, appear in breast milk, and some have caused adverse reactions in infants. They can be divided into two categories: combination and progestin-only. The combination products contain estrogen, which has been implicated in adverse reactions in infants and has been shown to decrease lactation. Although modern combination products have lower doses of estrogen than previous products, they are still best avoided during lactation. If you must use hormonal contraception, progestin-only products such as *norethindrone (Micronor, Nor-Q.D.)* and *norgestrel (Ovrette)* are preferable.

*Progesterone.* This natural hormone is sometimes given in suppositories for premenstrual syndrome. Amounts in milk are small and are not absorbed by the infant.

*Thyroid.* Thyroid products have one major, valid use—to replace thyroid hormone that is lacking in the bloodstream. When proper doses are taken, thyroid levels approximate those found in normal persons. Thyroid replacement therefore, poses no risks to the breastfed infant. Large daily doses of thyroid hormone (over 120 milligrams of thyroid or 0.2 milligrams of *levothyroxine*), as occasionally used in diet therapy, may pose a hazard to the infant as well as to the mother.

*Antithyroid agents.* Two types of agents are available. The most commonly used is *propylthiouracil.* Recent data indicate that, with due caution, breastfeeding during treatment with this drug is safe.

The other type of antithyroid drug is represented by the agents *methimazole* and *carbimazole.* It appears that significant quantities of these drugs appear in milk and can be dangerous to the infant. They should not be used while breastfeeding.

*Insulin.* Insulin therapy for diabetes mellitus is like thyroid replacement in that it restores that which is missing. Any insulin entering the milk will not be absorbed into the infant's bloodstream, because insulin is inactivated in the stomach.

**Psychotherapeutic agents.** With most of these agents little is known about their excretion into milk or their effects on infants. Undertake nursing with caution if you are using one of these drugs.

*Major tranquilizers.* These drugs include the *phenothiazines,* such as *chlorpromazine, thioridazine, trifluoperazine, perphenazine,* and *fluphenazine;* the closely related *thioxanthines,* such as *thiothixene;* and the *butyrophenones,* such as *haloperidol.* It is known that small amounts of these drugs appear in breast milk, and occasionally they have caused drowsiness in breastfed infants. Long-term effects on the infant are not well known; however, there is currently no evidence that the small amounts excreted into milk are harmful.

*Antidepressants.* Tricyclic antidepressants, such as *amitriptyline, imipramine,* and *doxepin,* have been measured in breast milk, but there is still controversy about what these small levels do to the infant. No serious effects have yet been reported. Newer antidepressants such as *trazodone, maprotiline,* and *amoxapine* have been even less well studied, so no judgment can be made on their safety. The newest agent, *fluoxetine (Prozac),* is very long-acting, has an even longer-acting metabolite, and should not be used while nursing. Older monoamine oxidase inhibitors, such as *phenelzine* and *tranylcypromine,* are very potent drugs and should not be used while breastfeeding.

*Lithium.* This drug reaches breast milk in significant levels and can accumulate in the bloodstream of the premature or newborn infant. An infant may show symptoms of lithium poisoning on becoming dehydrated due to diarrhea or a viral illness. A healthy infant may be breastfed during lithium therapy, but careful monitoring of the infant—including, perhaps, lithium blood level measurements—is essential. Stop breastfeeding if the infant becomes ill for any reason.

**Sedatives and sleep medications.** Several classes of drugs are included in this category. Although all of them can make an infant drowsy, some are more likely to do so than others. The drugs also differ in their duration of action, which affects their tendency to accumulate in the infant.

*Barbiturates.* Drugs in this class include *secobarbital, pentobarbital, phenobarbital, amobarbital,* and others. All may occasionally cause drowsiness in the breastfed infant, but none are particularly hazardous to the infant.

*Benzodiazepines.* Of all drugs, these are currently the most frequently used. They include *diazepam, chlordiazepoxide, flurazepam, triazolam,* and *alprazolam.* Although these drugs are safe in adults, infants do not readily metabolize them. They accumulate in the infant's body, causing drowsiness and, in some cases, interference with the binding of bilirubin in the bloodstream. Infant dependence and withdrawal have been reported with *alprazolam (Xanax).* All of these problems are accentuated in premature and newborn babies. Nursing mothers should generally use alternative drugs.

*Chloral hydrate.* Though old, this drug is still used. It has caused drowsiness in infants, but is safe for occasional use.

*Over-the-counter sleep medications.* These are *antihistamines;* the general precautions for antihistamines apply. (See Cough, Cold, Allergy, and Asthma Medications).

**Vaccines and skin tests.** Killed vaccines, as well as skin tests such as the one for tuberculosis *(PPD),* pose no known hazard to the breastfed infant. Examples of killed vaccines are tetanus, diphtheria-tetanus, hepatitis B, injectable polio, and some influenza vaccines. Live vaccines can be transmitted through breast milk, but do not endanger the baby. They include measles, mumps, rubella, oral polio, and influenza vaccines.

**Radiologic diagnostic agents.** A number of compounds are used in the radiologic diagnosis of various conditions. These compounds fall into two categories: radio-opaque contrast agents and radioactive agents. Consult the radiologist administering these tests who will usually have guidelines on breastfeeding with the specific agents. Simple X-rays of the mother's teeth or broken bones pose no hazards to the breastfed infant.

*Radio-opaque agents.* These are generally compounds that contain iodine, but they vary in the amount of iodine that can pass into milk. Many have no free iodine and therefore pose little risk to the infant. Others require a washout period of several hours after use.

*Radioactive agents.* Breastfeeding must be stopped for a time after these agents are administered. The period of time varies depending on the agent and the dose given; consult your radiologist for a specific recommendation. After exposure to some of these agents your body may give off significant amounts of radiation, particularly at close range. This means that not only will you have to stop breastfeeding, but you may not be able to hold your baby for a given period of time, since doing so would expose him to significant radiation.

**Recreational drugs.** These are drugs that are used for nontherapeutic purposes. Since they are not essential to the well-being of the mother, and their effects on the infant are often not known, their use is generally discouraged.

*Alcohol.* Alcohol readily passes into the milk. Large amounts of alcoholic beverages consumed over a short time can make a baby drunk and can inhibit lactation. Daily drinking by an alcoholic breastfeeding mother can lead to hormonal imbalances in the infant. Small to moderate amounts of alcohol used daily or nearly every day while nursing appear to cause delayed muscular development and coordination in infants, with the severity related to the amount of alcohol used. An occasional alcoholic beverage probably does not pose a serious danger to the infant, but waiting one hour per drink before nursing may provide an extra measure of safety.

*Caffeine.* Low to moderate intake of beverages containing caffeine is unlikely to cause problems in the infant, since the amount of caffeine that reaches the milk is usually not great. But very high caffeine intake can cause jitteriness and agitation in the infant.

*Cocaine.* Cocaine is an extremely toxic drug in infants because of their inability to metabolize it. Extreme agitation and crying is often noted in breastfed infants of cocaine users, and convulsions and death have occasionally been seen. Cocaine use while nursing is strongly discouraged. Breastfeeding should be discontinued for 24 to 48 hours after using cocaine.

*Marijuana.* There are few reports of the effects of marijuana in human infants who are breastfed. With a single use, levels in milk are apparently quite low, but the active component of the drug is very fat-soluble and can build up in the body with chronic use. It is likely that levels in milk would also be high after chronic use, because milk has a high fat content. Note, too, that an infant in the same room with the smoker will breathe in significant quantities of marijuana. Animal studies indicate that marijuana may suppress lactation.

*Phencyclidine (PCP).* Large amounts of this drug have been measured in breast milk. PCP should particularly be avoided during breastfeeding.

*Narcotics.* Large doses can cause narcotic effects and addiction in breastfed infants. Narcotic addicts should not breastfeed.

*Hallucinogens.* Information is lacking on the effects of these drugs during breastfeeding; however, levels in milk should be low by the time the mother has stopped feeling the effects of the drug.

*Tobacco.* Nicotine from smoking tobacco appears in breast milk. Though studies haven't proven it, other substances in smoke probably reach the milk as well. It should also be noted that an infant in the same room as the smoker will breathe in significant quantities of nicotine and other contaminants.

## Index to Common Drugs

Each brand name is listed in capital letters; the corresponding generic name is given after it. All generic names that do not appear as headings in the text are followed here by cross-references to the relevant sections. The names of combination products are followed by lists of the ingredients they contain; see the separate entry for each ingredient. Not all brands are listed, so if you can't find the name of a particular product in this list, look under the generic name of its ingredient or ingredients.

A-200: synergized pyrethrins. *See* scabicides and pediculocides

Accutane: isotretinoin. *See* acne products

acebutolol. *See* beta blockers

Achromycin: tetracycline

Adalat: nifedipine. *See* calcium channel blockers

Advil: ibuprofen. *See* nonsteroidal anti-inflammatory agents

Adriamycin: doxorubicin. *See* immunosuppressive agents

Afrin. *See* decongestants

Aldactazide: contains hydrochlorothiazide and spironolactone

Aldactone: spironolactone

Aldomet: methyldopa

Alkeran: melphalan. *See* immunosuppressive agents

aloe. *See* absorbable cathartics

alprazolam. *See* benzodiazepines

Amcill: ampicillin. *See* penicillins

Amikin: amikacin. *See* aminoglycosides

aminophylline. *See* theophylline

amitriptyline. *See* antidepressants

amoxapine. *See* antidepressants

Amoxil: amoxicillin. *See* penicillins

Anaprox: naproxen. *See* nonsteroidal anti-inflammatory agents

Apresoline: hydralazine

Asendin: amoxapine. *See* antidepressants

Atarax: hydroxyzine. *See* antihistamines

atenolol. *See* beta blockers

Ativan: lorazepam. *See* benzodiazepines

Augmentin: contains amoxicillin and clavulanate. *See* penicillins

azathioprine. *See* immunosuppressive agents

Azlin: azlocillin. *See* penicillins

Bactocil: oxacillin. *See* penicillins

Bactrim: contains sulfamethoxazole and trimethoprim. *See* sulfonamides

beclomethasone. *See* corticosteroids

Beclovent: beclomethasone. *See* corticosteroids

Beconase: beclomethasone. *See* corticosteroids

Benzac: benzoyl peroxide. *See* acne products

benzoyl peroxide. *See* acne products

Bicillin: penicillin G benzathine. *See* penicillins

BiCNU: carmustine. *See* immunosuppressive agents

birth control pills. *See* oral contraceptives

Bisthmuth subsalicylate. *See* antidiarrheals

Blenoxane: bleomycin. *See* immunosuppressive agents

bleomycin. *See* immunosuppressive agents

Blocadren: timolol. *See* beta blockers

bupivicaine. *See* local anesthetics

busulfan. *See* immunosuppressive agents

Butazolidin: phenylbutazone. *See* nonsteroidal anti-inflammatory agents

Cafergot: contains ergotamine and caffeine

Calan: verapamil. *See* calcium channel blockers

Capoten: captopril. *See* ACE inhibitors

captopril. *See* ACE inhibitors

Carafate: sucralfate

Cardizem: diltiazem. *See* calcium channel blockers.

carmustine. *See* immunosuppressive agents

cascara. *See* absorbable cathartics

CeeNU: lomustine. *See* immunosuppressive agents

Cerubidine: daunorubicin. *See* immunosuppressive agents

chlorambucil. *See* immunosuppressive agents

Chloraseptic. *See* cough, cold, allergy, and asthma medications

chlordiazepoxide. *See* benzodiazepines

Chloromycetin: chloramphenicol

chlorpheniramine. *See* antihistamines

chlorpromazine. *See* major tranquilizers

Chlor-Trimeton: chlorpheniramine. *See* antihistamines
Cipro: ciprofloxacin. *See* quinolones
ciprofloxacin. *See* quinolones
cisplatin. *See* immunosuppressive agents
clindamycin. *See* acne products
Clinoril: sulindac. *See* nonsteroidal anti-inflammatory agents
Cloxapen: cloxacillin. *See* pencillins
codeine. *See* narcotics
Colace: docusate. *See* nonabsorbable laxatives
contraceptives. *See* oral contraceptives
Corgard: nadolol. *See* beta blockers
cortisone. *See* corticosteroids
Cosmegen: dactinomycin. *See* immunosuppressive agents.
cyclophosphamide. *See* immunosuppressive agents
cytarabine. *See* immunosuppressive agents
Cytosar: cytarabine. *See* immunosuppressive agents
Cytoxan: cyclophosphamide. *See* immunosuppressive agents

dacarbazine. *See* immunosuppressive agents
dactinomycin. *See* immunosuppressive agents
Dalmane: flurazepam. *See* benzodiazepines
danthron. *See* absorbable cathartics
Darvon: propoxyphene. *See* narcotics
daunorubicin. *See* immunosuppressive agents
Decadron: dexamethasone. *See* corticosteroids
Declomycin: demeclocycline. *See* tetracyclines
Demerol: meperidine. *See* narcotics
Depakene: valproic acid
Depakote: valproic acid
Desquam-X: benzoyl peroxide. *See* acne products
Desyrel: trazodone. *See* antidepressants
dexamethasone. *See* corticosteroids
diazepam. *See* benzodiazepines
diclofenac. *See* nonsteroidal anti-inflammatory agents
DiGel. *See* antacids.
Dilantin. *See* phenytoin
diltiazem. *See* calcium channel blockers
diphenoxylate. *See* antidiarrheals
divalproex. *See* valproic acid
Dolobid: diflunisal. *See* nonsteroidal anti-inflammatory agents

doxepin. *See* antidepressants
doxorubicin. *See* immunosuppressive agents
Dyazide: contains hydrochlorothiazide
Dynapen: dicloxacillin. *See* penicillins

Elavil: amitriptyline. *See* antidepressants
Elimite: permethrin. *See* scabicides and pediculocides
enalapril. *See* ACE inhibitors
ephedrine. *See* decongestants
Ergomar: ergotamine
ergonovine: *See* ergot drugs
Ergostat: ergotamine
Ergotrate: ergonovine. *See* ergot drugs
Esidrix: hydrochlorothiazide.
etoposide. *See* immunosuppressive agents

famotidine. *See* histamine H-2 antagonists
Feldene: piroxicam. *See* nonsteroidal anti-inflammatory agents
Fibercon. *See* nonabsorbable laxatives
Flagyl: metronidazole
flunisolide. *See* corticosteroids
fluorouracil. *See* immunosuppressive agents
fluoxetine. *See* antidepressants.
fluphenazine. *See* major tranquilizers
flurazepam. *See* benzodiazepines
Furadantin: nitrofurantion.
Furoxone: furazolidone

Gantanol: sulfamethoxazole. *See* sulfonamides
Gantrisin: sulfisoxazole. *See* sulfonamides
Garamycin: gentamicin. *See* aminoglycosides
Gelusil. *See* antacids
Geocillin: carbenicillin. *See* penicillins
Geopen: carbenicillin. *See* penicillins
Gynergen: ergotamine

Halcion: triazolam. *See* benzodiazepines
Haldol: haloperidol. *See* major tranquilizers
haloperidol. *See* major tranquilizers
Hydrocodone. *See* narcotics
HydroDiuril: hydrochlorothiazide
hydroxyzine. *See* antihistamines
Hygroton: chlorthalidone

imipramine. *See* antidepressants
Imodium: loperamide. *See* antidiarrheals
Imuran: azathioprine. *See* immunosuppressive agents
Inderal: propranolol. *See* beta blockers

Indocin: indomethacin. *See* nonsteroidal anti-inflammatory agents
INH. *See* isoniazid
Iodinated glycerol. *See* cough medicines
Isoptin: verapamil. *See* calcium channel blockers

Kao-Pectate: kaolin-pectin. *See* antidiarrheals
Kwell: lindane. *See* scabicides and pediculocides

Labetalol. *See* beta blockers
Lanoxin: digoxin
Larotid: amoxicillin. *See* penicillins
Lasix: furosemide
Leukeran: chlorambucil. *See* immunosuppressive agents
Librium: chlordiazepoxide. *See* benzodiazepines
lidocaine. *See* local anesthetics
lomustine. *See* immunosuppressive agents
loperamide. *See* antidiarrheals
Lopressor: metoprolol. *See* beta blockers
lorazepam. *see* benzodiazepines
Ludiomil: maprotiline. *See* antidepressants

Maalox. *See* antacids
Macrodantin: nitrofurantoin
maprotiline. *See* antidepressants
Marcaine: bupivicaine. *See* local anesthetics
Matulane: procarbazine. *See* immunosuppressive agents
Meclomen: meclofenamate. *See* nonsteroidal anti-inflammatory agents
Mellaril: thioridazine. *See* major tranquilizers
melphalan. *See* immunosuppressive agents
meperidine. *See* narcotics
mercaptopurine. *see* immunosuppressive agents
Metamucil. *See* nonabsorbable laxatives
methadone. *See* narcotics
Methergine. methylergonovine. *See* ergot drugs
methotrexate.*See* immunosuppressive agents
methylergonovine. *See* ergot drugs
metoprolol. *See* beta blockers
Mexate: methotrexate. *See* immunosuppressive agents
Mezlin: mezlocillin. *See* penicillins
milk of magnesia. *See* nonabsorbable laxatives

Minocin: minocycline. *See* tetracyclines
Mithracin: mithramycin. *See* immunosuppressive agents
mithramycin. *See* immunosuppressive agents
mitomycin. *See* immunosuppressive agents
morphine. *See* narcotics
Motrin: ibuprofen. *See* nonsteroidal anti-inflammatory agents
Mutamycin: mitomycin. *See* immunosuppressive agents
Mylanta. *See* antacids
Myleran: busulfan. *See* immunosuppressive agents
Mysoline: primidone

nadolol. *See* beta blockers
Nalfon: fenoprofen. *See* nonsteroidal anti-inflammatory agents
Naprosyn: naproxen. *See* nonsteroidal anti-inflammatory agents
Nardil: phenelzine. *See* antidepressants
Nasalide: flunisolide. *See* corticosteroids
Navane: thiothixene. *See* major tranquilizers
Netromycin: netilmicin. *See* aminoglycosides
nifedipine. *See* calcium channel blockers
nitrous oxide. *See* general anesthetics
nizatidine. *See* histamine H-2 antagonists
Noctec: chloral hydrate
norethindrone: *See* oral contraceptives
norethynodrel: *See* oral contraceptives
norfloxacin. *See* quinolones
Normodyne: labetalol. *See* beta blockers
Noroxin: norfloxacin. *See* quinolones.
Novocaine: procaine. *See* local anesthetics
Nuprin: ibuprofen. *See* nonsteroidal anti-inflammatory agents

Omnipen: ampicillin. *See* penicillins
Oncovin: vincristine. *See* immunosuppressive agents
Oretic: hydrochlorothiazide
Organidin: iodinated glycerol. *See* cough medicines
oxacillin. *See* penicillins
oxazepam. *See* benzodiazepines
oxy stoxy 10: benzoyl peroxide. *See* acne products.

Parnate: tranylcypromine. *See* antidepressants
Pen Vee K: penicillin V. *See* penicillins
Pepto-Bismol: bisthmuth subsalicylate. *See* antidiarrheals

Percocet. *See* narcotics
Percodan. *See* narcotics
permethrin: *See* Scabicides and pediculocides
perphenazine. *See* major tranquilizers
phenazopyridine: *See* sulfonamides
phenelzine. *See* antidepressants
phenylpropanolamine. *See* decongestants
Phospho-Soda. *See* nonabsorbable laxatives
pindolol. *See* beta blockers
Pipracil: piperacillin. *See* penicillins
Platinol: cisplatin. *See* immunosuppressive agents
Polycillin: ampicillin. *See* penicillins
Polymox: amoxicillin. *See* penicillins
Principen: ampicillin. *See* penicillins
Procardia: nifedipine. *See* calcium channel blockers
Prolixin: fluphenazine. *See* major tranquilizers
Pronestyl: procainamide
propoxyphene. *See* narcotics
propranolol. *See* beta blockers
propylthiouracil. *See* antithyroid agents
Prostaphlin: oxacillin. *See* penicillins
Prozac: fluoxetine. *See* antidepressants
pseudoephedrine. *See* decongestants
PTU: propylthiouracil. *See* antithyroid agents
Purinethol: mercaptopurine. *See* immunosuppressive agents
Pyridium: *See* sulfonamides

ranitidine. *See* histamine H-2 antagonists
Retin-A: tretinoin. *See* acne products
Rid: synergized pyrethrins. *See* scabicides and pediculocides
Riopan. *See* antacids
Rolaids. *See* antacids
Rondomycin: methacycline. *See* tetracyclines

Sandimmune: cyclosporine. *See* immunosuppressive agents
Sectral: acebutolol. *See* beta blockers
senna. *See* absorbable cathartics
Sensorcaine: bupivicaine. *See* local anesthetics
Septra: contains sulfamethoxazole and trimethoprim. *See* sulfonamides
Serax: oxazepam. *See* benzodiazepines
Sinequan: doxepin. *See* antidepressants
Slo-Bid: theophylline
Slo-Phyllin: theophylline
Spectrobid: bacampicillin. *See* penicillins
SSKI: iodide. *See* cough products

Stelazine: trifluoperazine. *See* major tranquilizers
Sucrets. *See* cough, cold, allergy, and asthma medications
Sudafed: pseudoephedrine. *See* decongestants
Sumycin: tetracycline

Tagamet: cimetidine
Tapazole: methimazole. *See* antithyroid agents
Tegopen: cloxacillin. *See* penicillins
Tegretol: carbamazepine
Tenormin: atenolol. *See* beta blockers
Terramycin: oxytetracycline
Tetrex: tetracycline. *See* tetracyclines
Theo-dur: theophylline
thioguanine: *See* immunosuppressive agents
thioridazine. *See* major tranquilizers
thiothixene. *See* major tranquilizers
Thorazine: chlorpromazine. *See* major tranquilizers
Ticar: ticarcillin. *See* penicillins
Timentin: contains ticarcillin and clavulanate. *See* penicillins
timolol. *See* beta blockers
Tobrex: tobramycin. *See* aminoglycosides
Tofranil: imipramine. *See* antidepressants
Tolectin: tolmetin. *See* nonsteroidal anti-inflammatory agents
Trandate: labetalol. *See* beta blockers
tranylcypromine. *See* antidepressants
trazodone. *See* antidepressants
tretinoin. *See* acne products
triamcinolone. *See* corticosteroids
triazolam. *See* benzodiazepines
trifluoperazine. *See* major tranquilizers
Trilafon: perphenazine. *See* major tranquilizers
Tums. *See* antacids
Tylenol: acetaminophen

Unipen: nafcillin. *See* penicillins

Valium: diazepam. *See* benzodiazepines
Vancenase: beclomethasone. *See* corticosteroids
Vanceril: beclomethasone. *See* corticosteroids
Vasotec: enalapril. *See* ACE inhibitors
V Cillin K: penicillin V. *See* penicillins
Vectrin: minocycline. *See* tetracyclines
Velban: vinblastine. *See* immunosuppressive agents
VePesid: etoposide. *See* immunosuppressive agents

Verapamil. *See* calcium channel blockers

Versapen: hetacillin. *See* penicillins

Vibramycin: doxycycline. *See* tetracyclines

Vicodin: contains hydrocodone. *See* narcotics

vinblastine. *See* immunosuppressive agents

vincristine. *See* immunosuppressive agents

Visken: pindolol. *See* beta blockers

Vistaril: hydroxyzine. *See* antihistamines

Voltaren: diclofenac. *See* nonsteroidal anti-inflammatory agents

Wycillin: penicillin G procaine. *See* penicillins

Xanax: alprazolam. *See* benzodiazepines

Xylocaine: lidocaine. *See* local anesthetics

Zantac: ranitidine. *See* cimetidine

Zovirax: acyclovir

# Selected References

American Academy of Pediatrics. *Report on the Assessment of Scientific Evidence Relating to Infant-Feeding Practices and Infant Health. Pediatrics* 74 (1984).

Auerbach, Kathleen G. "Employed Breastfeeding Mothers: Problems They Encounter." *Birth* 11 (1984): 17–20.

Auerbach, Kathleen G., and Gartner, Laurence. "Breastfeeding and Human Milk: Their Association with Jaundice in the Neonate." *Clinics in Perinatology* 14 (1987), 89–107.

Auerbach, Kathleen G., and Guss, E. "Maternal Employment and Breastfeeding: A Study of 567 Women's Experiences." *American Journal of Disease in Childhood* 138 (1984): 958–60.

Boggs, Kathleen R., and Rau, Penny K. "Breastfeeding the Premature Infant." *American Journal of Nursing* 83 (1983): 1437–39.

Brewster, Dorothy Patricia. *You Can Breastfeed Your baby . . . Even in Special Situations.* Emmaus, Penn.: Rodale Press, 1979.

Brown, Marie Scott, and Hurlock, Joan T. "Preparation of the Breast for Breastfeeding." *Nursing Research* 24 (1975): 448–51.

Bumgarner, Norma Jane. *Mothering Your Nursing Toddler.* Franklin Park, Ill.: La Leche League International, 1982.

Copeland, Cynthia A., Raebel, Marsha A., and Wagner, Sheldon L. "Pesticide Residue in Lanolin." *Journal of the American Medical Association* 261 (1989): 242.

DeCarvalho, M., Hall, M., and Harvey, D. "Effects of Water Supplementation on Physiological Jaundice in Breast-fed Babies." *Archives of Disease in Childhood* 56 (1981): 568–69.

Ehrenkranz R., and Ackerman, B. "Metoclopromide Effect on Faltering Milk Production by Mothers of Premature Infants." *Pediatrics* 78 (1986): 614–20.

Frantz, Kittie B. "Techniques for Successfully Managing Nipple Problems and the Reluctant Nurser in the Early Postpartum Period." In *Human Milk, Its Biological and Social Value*, edited by S. Frier. Amsterdam: Exerpta Medica, 1980.

Frantz, Kittie B., Fleiss, Paul M., and Lawrence, Ruth A. "Management of the Slow-Gaining Breastfed Baby." *Keeping Abreast Journal* 3 (1978): 287–308.

Friedland, G., and Klein R. "Transmission of the Human Immunodeficiency Virus." *New England Journal of Medicine* 317 (1987): 1125–35.

Goldfarb, Johanna, and Tibbetts, Edith. *Breastfeeding Handbook.* Hillside, N.J.: Enslow Publishers, 1980.

Health Education Associates. *Nursing and Weaning the Older Baby and Toddler.* Willow Grove, Penn.: Health Education Associates, 1978.

Health Education Associates. *Weaning Your Breastfed Baby.* Willow Grove, Penn.: Health Education Associates, 1978.

La Leche League International. *The Womanly Art of Breastfeeding.* Franklin Park, Ill.: La Leche League International, 1981.

Lawrence, Ruth A. *Breastfeeding: A Guide for the Medical Profession.* St. Louis: C. V. Mosby, 1980.

Lowman, Kaye. *Of Cradles and Careers: A Guide to Reshaping Your Job to Include a Baby in Your Life.* Franklin Park, Ill.: La Leche League International, 1984.

Meier, Paula. "A Program to Support Breastfeeding in the High-Risk Nursery." *Perinatology/Neonatology* 4 (1980): 43–48.

Meier, Paula. *Breastfeeding Your Special-Care Baby.* Chicago: Michael Reese Hospital Publications, 1980.

Meier, Paula, and Anderson, G. "Responses of Small Preterm Infants to Bottle- and Breast-feeding." *Maternal-Child Nursing* 12 (1987): 97–105.

Michigan Department of Public Health, *Minutes of the Panel on Recommendations Relating to PBB and Nursing Mothers,* 1976.

Price, Anne, and Bamford, Nancy. *The Breastfeeding Guide for the Working Woman.* New York: Wallaby Books, 1983.

Pryor, Karen. *Nursing Your Baby.* New York: Pocket Books, 1973.

Raphael, Dana. *The Tender Gift: Breast Feeding.* New York: Schocken, 1976.

Riordan, Janice. *A Practical Guide to Breastfeeding.* St. Louis: C. V. Mosby, 1983.

Riordan, Janice, and Nichols, Francine. "A Descriptive Study of Lactation Mastitis in Long-term Breastfeeding Women." *Journal of Human Lactation* 6, no. 2: 53–58.

Rozdilsky, Mary Lou, and Banet, Barbara. *What Now? A Handbook for New Parents.* New York: Charles Scribner's Sons, 1975.

Satter, Ellyn. *Child of Mine: Feeding with Love and Good Sense.* Expanded ed. Palo Alto, Calif.: Bull Publishing, 1986.

Weintraub, R., Hams, G., Meerkin M., and Rosenberg, A. "High Aluminum Content of Infant Milk Formulas." *Archives of Disease in Childhood* 61 (1986): 914–16.

Wickizer, Thomas M., Brilliant, Lawrence B., Copeland, Richard., and Tilden, Robert. "Polychlorinated Biphenyl Contamination of Nursing Mothers' Milk in Michigan." *American Journal of Public Health* 71 (1981): 132–37.

Woolridge, M. W., and Fisher, Chloe. "Colic, 'Overfeeding,' and Symptoms of Lactose Malabsorption in the Breast-fed Baby: A Possible Artifact of Feed Management?" *The Lancet* 2(1988): 382–84.

# Suggested Supplemental Reading

Most of the books listed here are generally available in bookstores. If you can't find them locally, contact Birth and Life Bookstore, ICEA Bookcenter, or NAPSAC Mail Order Bookstore, all of which publish catalogs. Birth and Life Bookstore and ICEA Bookcenter accept telephone orders.

Birth and Life Bookstore
P.O. Box 70625
Seattle, Washington 98107
206-789-4444
800-736-0631 (orders only)

NAPSAC Mail Order Bookstore
P.O. Box 267
Marble Hill, Missouri 63764

ICEA Bookcenter
P.O. Box 20048
Minneapolis, Minnesota 55420
612-854-8660
800-624-4934 (orders only)

La Leche League pamphlets are available by contacting—

La Leche League International, Inc.
9616 Minneapolis Avenue
Franklin Park, Illinois 60131
312-455-7730

Anderson, Kathryn. *Nursing Your Adopted Baby.* Franklin Park, Ill.: La Leche League International, 1983.

This pamphlet is available for $1.95 from La Leche League. Ask for publication 55.

Avery, Jimmie Lynne. *A Brief Discussion of Adoptive Nursing: An Introduction to the Topic.* Athens, Tenn.: Lact-Aid International, 1972.

This pamphlet is available free of charge from Lact-Aid International, P.O. Box 1066, Athens, Tenn. 37303.

Danner, Sarah Coulter, and Cerutti, Edward R. *Nursing Your Neurologically Impaired Baby.* Rochester, N.Y.: Childbirth Graphics, 1984.

For a copy of this pamphlet, send $.50 to Childbirth Graphics, P.O. Box 17025, Irondequoit Post Office, Rochester, N.Y. 14617-0325.

Fraiberg, Selma H. *The Magic Years*. New York: Charles Scribner's Sons, 1959.

A classic text on child development from infancy to six years.

Good, Judy. *The Diabetic Mother and Breastfeeding*. Franklin Park, Ill.: La Leche League International, 1983.

La Leche League publication 17, this pamphlet is available for $.50.

Good, Judy. *Breastfeeding the baby with Down's Syndrome*. Franklin Park, Ill.: La Leche League International, 1985.

La Leche League Publication 23. $.75.

Jones, Sandy. *Crying Baby, Sleepless Nights*. Boston: Harvard Common Press, 1992.

Robertson, Laurel, Flinders, Carol, and Godfrey, Bronwen. *The New Laurel's Kitchen*. Berkeley: Ten Speed Press, 1986.

Satter, Ellyn. *Child of Mine: Feeding with Love and Good Sense*. Expanded ed. Palo Alto, Calif.: Bull Publishing, 1986.

Thevenin, Tine. *The Family Bed: An Age Old Concept in Child Rearing*. Minneapolis: Tine Thevenin, 1976.

Available from Birth and Life Bookstore, ICEA Bookcenter, and La Leche League.

# Index

Cocoa butter, 50, 58
Colds, baby's, 113, 124
Colic, 115, 125–30
  and hyperlactation syndrome, 129
Colostrum, 25, 27, 39–40, 64, 70
  expressing, 28, 66
  and premature baby, 91, 92
Constipation, 69, 103, 114
  in mother, 79, 103, 105, 128, 155
Contraception, 157, 165, 198
Convenience of breastfeeding, 4, 5
Coolers, for storing breast milk, 150, 188
Counseling, 123. *See also* Support
Cramping, uterine, 48
Creams and lotions for breasts, 25, 27, 50, 58, 117
Crib death, 109
Cross-cuddle hold, 43, 57
Crying, 114, 125–30, 181
  intense, 114–15, 126–30
  *See also* Fussiness
*Crying Babies, Sleepless Nights* (Sandy Jones), 127
Cuddle hold, 42–43, 96
Cup, 141, 172
  drinking from, 148
  weaning to, 182
Cysts, in breast, 120

Dehydration, 113
Delivery
  cesarean, 43, 45, 46, 89, 103
  nursing after, 31, 39–40, 43, 45, 46
Depression, postpartum, 67–68, 104, 122–23
  coping measures for, 123
Developmental problems, baby with, 99–100
Diabetes, nursing mother with, 40, 59, 88–89
Diaper rash, 127
  thrush (yeast), 59, 119, 125, 127
Diapers, 34, 181
  wet, as sign of adequate milk intake, 49, 79, 114, 130–31
Diaper service, 34
Diarrhea, baby's, 113
Diaphragm, 157
Diet, baby's
  solid foods in, 158–61, 171–75
  toddler's, 176
  vegetarian, 173–74
Diet, mother's, 64, 155, 165, 170–71
  baby's reactions to, 108–9, 124–25, 128–29
  diabetic, 88–89

elimination, for allergic baby, 128–29
  for nursing twins, 97
  postpartum, 35, 51, 67, 105–9, 123
  during pregnancy, 96
  and refusal to nurse, 124–25, 128
  vegetarian, 107
  while working, 152
Dietary supplements
  for infant, 111–12, 128
  for mother, 97, 108, 128
Dieting, 5, 106, 155
Dimples in baby's cheeks, while nursing, 49, 74, 80, 94
Discreet nursing, 4–5, 136
Distractibility, baby's, when nursing, 158
Doctor, selecting baby's, 31–32
Down's syndrome, nursing baby with, 99, 100
Dripping milk, 48. *See also* Leaking milk
Drugs
  index of common, 202–6
  recreational, 201
  safety of, 85, 189–201
  *See also* Medications
"Dry-up" medication, 27, 88
Ducts, plugged, 89, 117–18, 120, 121, 163

Ear infections, 113, 158
Eczema, on nipples, 60
Eggs, 129, 173
Engorgement, 28, 41, 50–51, 54–55, 61, 117
  treatment for, 54–55
Environmental pollutants, and breast milk, 85
Epilepsy, nursing mother with, 89
Episiotomy, 67, 155
Estrogen, 156
Eucerin (breast cream), 58
Exercise, in postpartum period, 103, 105, 123
Expressing milk, 141–48, 151–52
  breast pumps for, 142–47
  manually, 142
  for premature baby, 91–93

*Family Bed, The: An Age Old Concept* (Tine Thevenin), 181
Family members, support from, 35, 67. *See also* Partner
Fatigue, postpartum, 67. *See also* Rest, importance of
Fever, baby's, 113
Financial savings with breastfeeding, 6

## Other books for the family
## from The Harvard Common Press

All are available by mail-order from The Harvard Common Press, 535 Albany Street, Boston, Massachusetts 02118. When ordering, please include a check for the price specified plus shipping and handling charges of $3.00 for a single book and $.50 for each additional book. If the order is to be sent to a Massachusetts address, add 5 percent sales tax.

THE BIRTH PARTNER:
EVERYTHING YOU NEED TO KNOW
TO HELP A WOMAN THROUGH CHILDBIRTH
by Penny Simkin, P.T.
$16.95 cloth     ISBN 1-55832-011-3
$8.95 paper     ISBN 1-55832-010-5

"Destined to become the birth partner's bible. We have needed something like this for a long, long time."—Marian Tompson, cofounder of La Leche League

"Penny Simkin shows how giving support in childbirth is not only a matter of helping a woman through labor and delivery—important though that is—but also of enabling her to cherish a meaningful memory of birth."—Sheila Kitzinger, author of *The Complete Book of Pregnancy and Childbirth*

TOUGH QUESTIONS:
TALKING STRAIGHT WITH YOUR KIDS
ABOUT THE REAL WORLD
by Sheila Kitzinger and Celia Kitzinger
$19.95 cloth     ISBN 1-55832-033-4
$12.95 paper     ISBN 1-55832-032-6

The Kitzingers frankly and sympathetically examine the questions that challenge today's parents—questions about money, justice, sex, violence, and religion, among other subjects. Instead of supplying pat answers, they help parents explore their own most important values so they can confidently pass on these values to their children.

HELPING CHILDREN COPE WITH SEPARATION AND LOSS
by Claudia L. Jewett
$14.95 cloth     ISBN 0-916782-27-1
$8.95 paper     ISBN 0-916782-53-0

A compassionate, practical book for any adult who wants to help a child recover from the stages of denial and mourning that follow the loss of a loved one, whether from a death, divorce, moving, hospitalization, or simply the politics of friendship.

"This is a book of warmth and wisdom, a resource for all caregivers to children in time of need."—*Publishers Weekly*

"A well-formulated, practical guide highly suitable for both laypersons and professionals."—*Library Journal*

ADOPTING THE OLDER CHILD
by Claudia L. Jewett
$9.95 paper     ISBN 0-916782-09-3

A family counselor and an adoptive parent, Jewett offers practical, understanding advice for every family considering adopting an older child.

"One of the truly fine books in its genre, rich with insights and practical counsel."
—*Publishers Weekly*

"Comprehensive and well-written. . . . not only a useful resource but enjoyable to read. A sensitive and realistic presentation."—*Social Work*

ACTIVE BIRTH:
THE NEW APPROACH TO GIVING BIRTH NATURALLY
by Janet Balaskas
$19.95 cloth     ISBN 1-55832-037-7
$12.95 paper     ISBN 1-55832-038-5

Balaskas helps women prepare for and experience a truly natural birth, whether at home or in the hospital. With exercises for before and after birth, and information about breathing, massage, and the best positions for labor and delivery.

"Janet Balaskas captures the psychological essence of giving birth and the spirit of active participation so important to a woman's self-esteem during pregnancy and delivery."—Gayle Peterson, author of *Birthing Normally* and *An Easier Childbirth*

A GOOD BIRTH, A SAFE BIRTH:
CHOOSING AND HAVING THE CHILDBIRTH EXPERIENCE YOU WANT
by Diana Korte and Roberta Scaer
$21.95 cloth     ISBN 1-55832-042-3
$12.95 paper     ISBN 1-55832-041-5

"Unless parents are aware of and *ask* for their options, they will receive the standardized high-risk medical care that minimizes the joy and dignity of childbirth. *A Good Birth, A Safe Birth* gives them the tools they need to get the birth experience they want and deserve."—Donna Ewy, author of *Preparation for Parenthood*

"A warm-hearted, level-headed, and devastatingly well-documented look at the way the medical world makes life miserable for women in childbirth. . . . Korte and Scaer tell you what to do to protect yourself *and* your baby from the unwanted interferences customary in most hospitals. . . . From now on I'm giving *A Good Birth, A Safe Birth* to all my pregnant friends."—Karen Pryor, author of *Nursing Your Baby*

EASING LABOR PAIN:
THE COMPLETE GUIDE TO A MORE COMFORTABLE AND
REWARDING BIRTH
by Adrienne B. Lieberman
$19.95 cloth     ISBN 1-55832-044-X
$10.95 paper     ISBN 1-55832-043-1

The only book devoted to the number one concern of expectant mothers. Ancient and modern techniques that work, for mothers, their partners, and their caregivers.

"Adrienne Lieberman is a childbirth educator, parent, and gifted writer. . . . Readers of this book will find her optimism and confidence contagious."—*Birth*

CRYING BABY, SLEEPLESS NIGHTS:
WHY YOUR BABY IS CRYING AND WHAT YOU CAN DO ABOUT IT
by Sandy Jones
$17.95 cloth     ISBN 1-55832-046-6
$8.95 paper     ISBN 1-55832-045-8

A reassuring, comprehensive guide to the many causes of baby crying. Helps parents determine what their baby's cries mean, and offers them practical suggestions for making their babies happier and for coping with their own emotions.

## Do you have a friend or relative who needs this book?

Just fill out a coupon below and we'll send it. Please make checks payable to the publisher, The Harvard Common Press. Send orders to:

> The Harvard Common Press
> 535 Albany Street
> Boston, Massachusetts 02118

— — — — — — — — — — — — — — — — — — — — — — — —

☐ Please send _____ copies of *The Nursing Mother's Companion,* @ $11.95 plus $3.00 postage and handling per book.

To _____
    name

At _____
    address

_____
city          state          zip

*Massachusetts residents add 5% sales tax.*

— — — — — — — — — — — — — — — — — — — — — — — —

☐ Please send _____ copies of *The Nursing Mother's Companion,* @ $11.95 plus $3.00 postage and handling per book.

To _____
    name

At _____
    address

_____
city          state          zip

*Massachusetts residents add 5% sales tax.*

— — — — — — — — — — — — — — — — — — — — — — — —